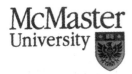

May 14, 2004

Dr. Blake Graham

Dear Blake

On behalf of all the staff, faculty members and researchers with whom you have collaborated in recent years, it is indeed my pleasure to acknowledge and thank you for your contribution to McMaster University and commend you on the publication of your book.

I appreciate the personal decision it was to make a generous donation in memory of your wife, Barbara. The joint donation to McMaster and The Ontario Veterinary College (OVC) created a unique and positive opportunity for research that would help identify specific kinds of cancers that are common among animals and humans and how they can be treated most effectively. Your inspiration and support provided the resources needed to further this important research being done by McMaster's Dr. Jack Gauldie, Chairman, Department of Pathology and Director of the Immunology Laboratory. Dr. Gauldie is world renowned for his leading edge research in cancer and we are most proud that he is a part of the McMaster team. It was indeed a pleasure for Dr. Gauldie to work in co-operation with the OVC representatives thereby creating the opportunity to combine both areas of specialty and expertise.

The results have been tremendous and continue to flourish. *The Barbara Graham Breast Cancer Research Fund* provided significant support for Dr. Gauldie's research and clinical trials dedicated to reducing the size of breast cancer tumours. As the research expanded with available funding, it also supported the need for new facilities that have since been built on campus to better accommodate this essential work. At OVC your support helped establish a laboratory dedicated to the study of cancer research in animals. The research results from both labs has created mutually beneficial outcomes that helps advance the extensive work being done to gain control over a frightening disease. You should be very proud to know that your foresight and generosity has allowed for major initiatives in the development of gene-based immunotherapy for breast cancer and encouraged related funding from other Canadian research agencies.

Congratulations on the publication of your memoirs, *Anecdotes From The Life of a Veterinarian,* which includes your touching story about your gift to McMaster and OVC. I commend you on your achievement, and I thank you sincerely for your kindness and support that will help improve the lives of many others around the world. I know Barbara would be very proud.

Yours sincerely,

Peter George,
President and Vice-Chancellor

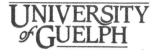

UNIVERSITY of GUELPH

OFFICE OF THE PRESIDENT

June 4, 2004

Dr. Blake Graham
6 Front Street North
Southampton, ON N0H 2L0

Dear Dr. Graham, Blake,

It is my great pleasure to express formally my thanks to you, a valued member of our alumni community for your creative leadership in supporting work in comparative medicine and doing so in a way that advances the University of Guelph's goals in this area. Your vision of comparative medicine as a key to addressing critical health issues and your willingness to marshall resources in support of its study, have inspired great appreciation for your work among the faculty, students and staff at the University of Guelph and McMaster University.

As a result of your establishment of the **Barbara Graham Cancer Research Fund** initiative 10 years ago, we have seen creative research partnership between U. of G.'s Ontario Veterinary College (OVC) and McMaster University. This collaboration continues to this day. Dr. Stephen Kruth, Professor, Small Animal Medicine at the OVC, often speaks of the inspiration your financial gift provided to his research on cancer in animals, and the benefits that have accrued from the related collaboration with his colleagues at McMaster. Dr. Kruth is internationally-recognized for his expertise in oncology and the Fund has played an important role in enabling the U. of G. to support his ground-breaking work.

Initially, Dr. Kruth's research focused on the progression of cancer in animals. Given that their cancer develops much more quickly than humans, studying animals afflicted with the disease offers useful insight into understanding tumour growth and behaviour. Over the years, the research studies have evolved and, as a result of what has been learned, we see direct benefits to treating cancer in both people and animals. The partner researchers from both institutions are now engaged in the development of therapeutic vaccines to treat cancer, with protocols being developed for use of the vaccine with humans and pets. This has the potential to offer a tremendous breakthrough for small animal medicine and human health care.

Your investment in cancer research created a bridge between two excellent institutions – each interested in advancing knowledge about human health from their unique perspectives. This partnership has served as a model for other wide-ranging collaborative investigations addressing

Dr. Blake Graham   June 4, 2004

issues affecting public health and animal care. Your vision and valued investment in the University of Guelph have been key catalysts in this regard.

In closing, I add warm congratulations to my thanks in light of the completion of your memoirs, **Anecdotes From The Life of a Veterinarian**, describing some of the experiences and perspectives that have underpinned your leadership and abiding vision about the role of comparative medicine in addressing human health challenges. On behalf of the University of Guelph, and particularly OVC, I am grateful for your inspiration and commitment to our research goals.

With very best wishes.

Yours sincerely,

Alastair J. S. Summerlee
President and Vice-Chancellor

SOW'S EAR
to
SILK PURSE

Anecdotes from the Life of a Veterinarian

J. E. B. Graham, DVM

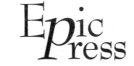

Epic Press

Belleville, Ontario, Canada

SOW'S EAR TO SILK PURSE

Copyright © 2004, J. E. B. Graham, DVM

Canadian Intellectual Property Office

Registration Number 1015943, October 30, 2003

Library and Archives Canada Cataloguing in Publication

Graham, J. E. B. (James Edward Blake), 1926-
    Sow's ear to silk purse / J.E.B. Graham.

    First ed. published Toronto : s.n., 2002 under title:Sow's ear - silk purse.
ISBN 1-55306-912-9.--ISBN 1-55306-914-5 (LSI ed.)

    1. Veterinarians--Canada--Biography. I. Graham, J. E. B. (James Edward Blake), 1926- . Sow's ear - silk purse. II. Title.

SF613.G72A3 2004   636.089'092   C2005-900653-6

Edited by Alain Lefevre

*All profits from the sales of this book
will be donated to the
Barbara Graham Breast Cancer Research Fund*

Epic Press is an imprint of *Essence Publishing*. For more information, contact:
20 Hanna Court, Belleville, Ontario, Canada K8P 5J2
Phone: 1-800-238-6376 • Fax: (613) 962-3055
E-mail: publishing@essencegroup.com • Internet: www.essencegroup.com

Printed in Canada
by

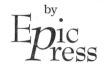

Dedication

*To the memory of my first love
and late wife, Barbara
To my second love, Joan, who
filled a great void in my life
To my daughter, Janet, a
competent family physician
And to my granddaughter, Carolyn,
who has the ability to be outstanding
in whatever she chooses
as a goal for her life.*

Contents

College Years

Veterinary Practice

Letters to Politicians

Acknowledgements

I am indebted to my second wife, Joan, who has been a source of strength in my later years. She also has my thanks for her assistance in editing this material. I am also indebted to Janet for her advice on the manuscript, to her husband Michael, to my stepson John Grainger and to Andrew Giles, son of my friends Ken and Sally Giles, for their computer advice and assistance. Thanks to Norman Wagner for permission to use a quotation from his article "Foot & Mouth Disease—A Regina Teenager's Memories" as well as part of our correspondence. In addition I would like to thank Mrs. Dorothy Roney, our next-door neighbour in Florida, for her help on the first manuscript.

Thanks are due to my editor, Mr. Alain Lefevre.

I also appreciate the help of my surgical mentor, Dr. James Archibald, for his assistance in editing these recollections. Jim graduated two years before me. During his senior year at the Ontario Veterinary College, Jim was associated with Dr. Jacob

13

Markowitz at the University of Toronto. Dr. Markowitz, a medical doctor, had written a textbook on experimental surgery and utilized animals to perfect new surgical procedures for humans. Jim's training under Dr. Markowitz convinced him that similar sterile procedures should be applied in veterinary surgery. When he started to teach in 1950, his first students were only a year behind him. Since he was known to most of them, it was obvious that they had to be convinced of the necessity for adopting his new theory. Until his retirement Jim was a professor at OVC, and he wrote many professional articles as well as veterinary textbooks on surgery. Most veterinary colleges eventually adopted his work on the necessity for sterile surgery in animals. Jim was one of the first in the world to stress the application of this subject in veterinary medicine.

I was recently informed that Dr. Archibald had passed away. I got further details in the following e-mail, dated January 3, 2005.

Hi Blake,

It was good speaking with you last night. After doing some digging, I found that Dr. Archibald's request was to NOT have any public notification of his passing. There was no visitation, and no service. This following is everything that I can find, taken from the OVC website. I'll follow up on the book.

Take care,

Steve

Dr. James Archibald, whose outstanding contributions to OVC and veterinary medicine as a whole are widely and internationally recognized, passed away on Saturday, December 11, in his 86th year. Dr. Archibald joined OVC as a faculty member after his graduation from the College in 1949, and continued in teaching and research until his retirement in 1986.

Acknowledgements

Dr. Archibald is regarded as a pioneer in the development of veterinary surgery. His work in this area markedly influenced both animal and human surgical techniques. He was editor of two editions of the text "Canine Surgery," one of the founders of the American College of Veterinary Surgery, and one of the first editors of the Canadian Veterinary Journal. At OVC, Dr. Archibald served the College and University in several roles. He was Chair of the Department of Clinical Studies, Director of Animal Care Services, Acting Associate Dean of Research, and member of the University Board of Governors. He was appointed University Professor Emeritus upon his retirement.

The honours and awards bestowed upon Dr. Archibald are many. In 1984, he was awarded the World Small Animal Veterinary Medical Association prize for scientific achievement. In 1990, the year he received the Order of Ontario, the Ontario Veterinary College Small Animal Clinic was named in his honour. In 2001, he was named OVC's Distinguished Alumnus.

Dr. Archibald was predeceased by his wife Hilda and is survived by three sons, Tom, John and David. His death is a profound loss to the veterinary community.

--

Stephen Kruth DVM, Dip ACVIM (Internal Medicine)
Professor
Department of Clinical Studies
University of Guelph

Preface

Be the Kind of Person Your Dog Thinks You Are

A friend gave us a gift of a set of drink coasters. Each had a different message, one of which was "Be the kind of person your dog thinks you are." An appropriate thought for a veterinarian's autobiography! I decided to borrow it as an underlying theme.

Rather than plagiarize the thoughts of someone else, I found the e-mail address of the distributor of the coasters, the Cedar Mountain Studio on Salt Spring Island, British Columbia, and sent the following message.

Cedar Mountain Studios:

I am a retired veterinarian currently doing a revision of a book that I published privately last year. The title of the book was Sow's Ear—Silk Purse; Anecdotes from the Life of a Veterinarian.

Recently I received a gift of some drink coasters with some intriguing messages. One in particular said: "Be kind of person that your dog thinks you are." I would like to use this message in my book and would be pleased to quote the source. Your reply would be appreciated.

Sincerely,

J.E.B. Graham DVM

The reply was as follows:

Hi Blake—Please go ahead and use that quote in your book. Don't worry about quoting me, because I heard it from a girlfriend in Toronto. My friend teaches a course on seven habits of highly effective people and other motivational topics. She said that part of the course was defining a quote or mantra that you want to live by. One of the men on the course said that it was his favorite quote and one that he wanted to live by. I don't think that this man was sure of the source either. Some quotes seem to be floating around. It is a fabulous one. Good luck with the book.

Susan Zacharias

Let us consider this quote. While it offers an admirable objective, I do not believe all dog owners live up to it. In some homes the dog is merely an ornament; in such case the compliment is not deserved.

Some dogs have hereditary mental defects, such as a vicious personality, and those dogs probably do not qualify to be a judge of their owner.

How about an owner who attempts to flaunt his affluence by bragging how much he paid for the dog? Since the dog could not be aware of the price paid for it, this could not have influenced his admiration of the owner.

Should an owner who has trained his or her dog to be an attack dog warrant such a compliment from the dog? Perhaps not. On the other hand, one wonders how many burglars through the ages have been chased away by barking dogs.

Many owners are very deserving of the admiration of their dogs. The seeing-eye dog creates a special partnership with its non-sighted owner. There are hearing-ear dogs, too, which can notify the handicapped owner that the baby is crying, or the doorbell is ringing, or the smoke detector has sounded. Owners of such animals form a lifetime partnership—man and dog, each dependent on the other. The dogs are often responsible for the very lives of their masters and for that reason are much appreciated. The dogs, much aware of their duties, thrive on the mutual bond. Most veterinarians, well aware of this relationship, provide service for these dogs at either no charge or greatly reduced fees.

There are other symbiotic man-dog relationships. Some dogs owned or handled by officers of police departments and by soldiers are trained for a specific purpose such as detecting narcotics or explosives. Some dogs are trained to assist their handlers on dangerous missions such as coping with armed thugs. In all of these situations, there is a synergy between the dog and its handler, and they greatly respect each other. These officers know that their lives may depend on their canine friends and treat them accordingly.

Doctors inform us that a canine companion can boost a stressed immune system and lower blood pressure. The presence of a dog, it has been insisted, can even suppress pain.

Are you the person your dog thinks you are? Have I been such a person? Perhaps my book will reveal the answer.

SECTION ONE

Youth

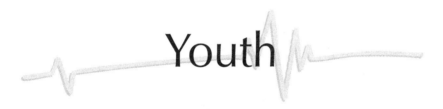

Chapter One

Family History

A brief family history is included since it has some relevance to later chapters. John Edward Blake Graham was born in the family residence, located on Lot 31, Concession 2, township of Dawn, county of Lambton, province of Ontario, on March 29, 1926. My sister and two brothers were also born in the family home, which is the present farmhouse. Built by my father in 1922, this house replaced the original log home in which my grandparents lived after they purchased the farm.

Family and friends knew this baby as Blake. I often wondered whether my parents thought I might be the last in the family and so gave me the remaining family first names. My mother's only brother was Blake Robertson. His first name came from his uncle, a Dr. Blake, who practised as a medical doctor in Michigan during the middle 1800s.

My mother, Mary Topping Robertson, was born and raised in the village of Oil Springs, Ontario. Her father bought a grocery store in the area soon after oil was discovered close to the village, the first such discovery in North America. She met her future husband when she taught at the one-room public school, S.S. (School Section) # 11, Dawn Township. The oil boom necessitated substantial growth in Oil Springs. Areas of growth included supplies for the oil fields and construction of rooming houses and hotels, as well as a great increase in the numbers of establishments devoted to the sale of alcoholic beverages.

My paternal grandfather, George, emigrated from England in 1875. His first wife died in the Old Country after the birth of her third child. His second marriage, to Margaret Baxter, was blessed with nine more children, five of whom were born in Canada. One can only speculate as to why George and Margaret were married. It would be reasonable to assume that George needed assistance to raise the small children and Margaret wanted to help and have her own family. In addition, while George was a poor tenant farmer, he was also a qualified land surveyor. Perhaps before being married they discussed moving to Canada where George's skills would be needed.

My father was the last of this second family. He was Edward Graham, nicknamed "Ed" as expected, and had no middle Christian name. All of the family first names may have been used, since he was the last of twelve children. The twelve offspring were listed by name and date of birth in the family Bible, which was the accepted means of recording births during that era. This Bible is still a valued family possession. My daughter Janet had the Bible professionally restored and is its custodian.

Upon arrival in Canada, George and Margaret lived on a farm in the township of Enniskillen several miles north of the present farm. On December 27, 1880, George purchased my birthplace from James King of Sarnia, Ontario. The purchase price for the farm was $423.00, which included a mortgage of $211.75. The farm has been designated as an Ontario Century Farm since the same family has owned it for more than a hundred years. The original shelter was a log cabin. Grandfather George, who had been a poor tenant farmer in England, cleared the land of trees so that a farming operation could be started. A relative had come to Canada some twenty years earlier, so George came by himself and stayed with this relative while he determined the feasibility of bringing his family to the new country. Deciding that the move was practical, he returned for the family. They sailed from Liverpool in 1875. His wife Margaret described the trip as a dreadful journey with "nothing to eat except porridge and potatoes."

As the family increased it became obvious that the farm was not able to generate enough income to support the large number of children. Most of the male offspring looked for greener fields and migrated to Minnesota and to British Columbia. My father went to Hibbing, Minnesota, where he joined some of his older brothers—John, David, George, Charles, and Joseph. Hibbing was a major producer of iron ore, which necessitated substantial activity in the construction industry. Edward was listed in the city directory of Hibbing of 1907 as a carpenter. He later moved to Vancouver and continued work as a carpenter until he returned to Lambton County to operate the family farm. Most of the girls in the family married local men and stayed in the area.

After purchasing the farm, Grandfather George started a construction company and directed his talents to road building and to the excavation of drainage ditches. Unfortunately he also developed a strong craving for alcohol and used much of his income to satisfy his habit.

After she was married, my mother found and kept most of the financial records related to the business of her in-laws. These records included the issuance and discharge of mortgages. The funds were used for payments to workmen employed by George in his construction business.

My Uncle Bill, two years older than my father, told me the following story: George had sold some sheep raised on the farm. He invited Bill to accompany him to spend the proceeds from the sale. They hitched up the horse and buggy for the eight-mile trip to the bustling village of Oil Springs. Two or three days later, the money to spend on booze exhausted, George raised his glass and toasted: "Well, Bill, here's to the last of the wee sheepies." Like his father, Bill developed a lifetime addiction to alcohol.

It is probable that my father recognized the problem of alcoholism, having observed his father and brother. He only on rare occasions had even one beer. The only time I know of that he had two beers on the same day took place the day I graduated from college and was invited to a stag party along with my father in celebration of my marriage to Barbara, which would take place the next day. It should be noted that the stag parties of 1951 were less boisterous than those of today.

After George died in 1920, my grandmother, Margaret, asked my father to come back from British Columbia to operate the family farm. He soon determined that the mortgages against the property exceeded its value. In spite of this he decided to stay to care for his widowed mother and try to save the homestead. Presumably to improve the cash flow and to help save the farm from its creditors, my grandmother and father decided to offer room and board to the local public school teacher. The farm was only one-quarter of a mile from the schoolhouse so was quite convenient for the teacher. My mother was the first teacher in the school to utilize the accommodation. My father fell in love with the new teacher. Probably my mother realized that my father was an honest hard-working man and that she could spend her years with him. He knew that she was a well-educated, intelligent, beautiful woman and chose her to be his wife. They were deeply in love for all of their married life.

They were married August 30, 1922. My older brother, Donald Robertson Graham, was born June 25, 1923. After my parents died, Donald owned and lived on the family farm until his passing on October 6, 2001. After Don passed away, title to the farm was transferred to my nephew Jim Graham, my brother Bill's son, leaving the title in the Graham name. As noted, I was the second child. The next child, my sister Margaret Yvonne Graham, was born February 6, 1928. Our youngest sibling, William Maurice Graham, was born on July 9, 1930. Bill died of heart failure in 1983. Grandmother Margaret lived with my parents until her death in 1923.

Chapter Two

Early Years of a Country Boy

My first memories go back to that period known later, but not then, as the Great Depression. While money was scarce during those years, our family had adequate food. My mother grew vegetables. There were farm animals, so we always had beef, pork, and poultry. The chickens provided eggs as well as meat. When the egg-laying ability of the hens diminished, we called them "cluckers," since they had lots of cackle and little egg production. But even the cluckers earned their feed, since they were willing to sit on a clutch of eggs produced by other hens until the surrogate eggs hatched. The rooster was still needed to fertilize the eggs being incubated by the cluckers. The maternal instincts of these old hens might remind the reader of certain grandmothers.

But when the elderly hen no longer served in the incubation of eggs, she became a candidate for the stew pot. Long cooking was necessary, since her meat would have been too tough to be considered for roast chicken. With long simmering and the addition of dumplings, a tasty meal came to be. Grandma Hen had done her best for mankind or, at least, for us!

When I think of chickens I am reminded of an incident that caused some laughter at our supper table one summer evening. My mother's sister Pearl and her husband Ferg had four children, the youngest of whom we called Doug. This lad spent most of the summers at the farm rather than at his home in Toronto. One evening mother had cooked a beef tongue, derived from a recently slaughtered steer. Father noticed that Doug was not eating his dinner with the usual gusto of a growing boy and asked if anything was wrong. Doug replied that he didn't like the thought of eating something that had rolled around in a steer's mouth. My father, with his usual droll humour, answered, "Doug, I noticed that you had no trouble eating two eggs this morning; where do you think they rolled around?"

At a very early age, perhaps four or five, I asked my father if the rooster had hurt the hen when he jumped on her. Dad assured me that he didn't. As I got a bit older I asked him about the bulls jumping on cows, the rams jumping on ewes, and, most amazing of all, I asked about the huge Percheron stallion mounting a mare. Since all of these occurrences took place within a few months of each other, Dad decided to explain. He told me about the planting of vegetables in mother's garden as well as the planting of wheat, oats and corn in the fields. He showed me acorns, hickory nuts, and walnuts and put them in the soil. He discussed how the plants and trees would grow. He then discussed how the ram, bull, stallion, and rooster were planting their seeds in order that new life could evolve. After the dissertation on agriculture and animal reproduction, he mentioned that human babies were conceived in the same way.

He spoke with simple dignity. I am not sure that I fully understood the biology lesson at the time, but I have never forgotten the lesson nor the good judgment with which it was offered.

When I remember those early years, it is now easy to appreciate the work and efforts of my parents in raising four children during the tough years of the depression. At that time children did not realize how hard their parents worked to look after their families. For example as well as planting and caring for the vegetable garden, my mother fed and watered the poultry, gathered the eggs, and cooked all of the meals. She helped with hand-milking the cows until the children were old enough to assist with this chore. When meats of various kinds were made ready for the winter meals, they had to be prepared by cooking into stews and canned for preservation. Some meats such as pork were salted down and kept in crocks in the cellar. Sides of beef were hung in an outdoor room in the late fall and preserved by freezing with pieces cut off as necessary for cooking on the wood stove. Farmers of today have electricity to freeze and preserve foods. It was not available in those days. My father also had his work consisting among other things of tilling the fields, harvesting the crops, supervising the health of the livestock, cleaning the stables and other jobs too numerous to mention. With all of these demands on natural human energy it is amazing that procreation could take place!

Chapter Three

The One-Room School

I began formal education at the age of five in the school known as SS # 11, township of Dawn, the school at which my mother had been the teacher prior to her marriage. There was only one teacher, who had to give instruction to all ages of children. In those days the classes were named "junior first," "senior first," through to "senior fourth," which was the equivalent of today's grade eight. The teacher normally began the day by giving lessons to the youngest children and then progressing to the oldest. Each child was assigned various tasks, and when these were completed the child could listen—and was expected to listen—to instruction being given to the older children. This excellent method of teaching allowed children with active minds to make rapid progress.

The teacher exerted strict discipline. If she deemed punishment more vigorous than scolding was necessary, she took a strap from her desk and applied a suitable number of strokes to the hands of the miscreant. The strap was more than an inch wide and was used when warranted—in my case, quite frequently. The teacher could have applied much more force had he or she so desired. Punishment normally took place at the front of the room where all of the students could see, very embarrassing to the recipient. If one of the students witnessing the punishment, which was always justified, broke out in laughter, that student was next in line for the same treatment.

The worst part of received the strap at school was an unwritten rule at our home that a repeat performance could be expected, usually with a bit more vigour. I have no criticism of such punishment provided that the feelings of the child are the only injury. I believe that I am a better person today because of the discipline.

My teachers said that I was a good listener who could quickly absorb new material. Accordingly the teacher moved me to new grades as she saw fit, which allowed me to finish public school at age eleven. In those days passing marks in a written examination set by the Province of Ontario were required for entrance to high school. This exam for students from various rural public schools in the area took place in the village of Oil Springs.

My parents considered that at eleven years of age I was too young to be sent to high school. We had no school buses for the transport of children from the farms to high schools in the adjacent towns. Arrangements for room and board had to be made with private homes. Suitable high schools were at least twelve miles away from our family farm. My mother, as a teacher herself, discussed various options with my teacher, Mr. Gordon Stinson, who taught at the local school. Mr. Stinson agreed to give me high school training as well as he could, a decision which was a great help to me. With the exception of French, he was able to provide reasonable instruction in high school subjects. My training by him lasted for two years in the one-room school.

Admitted to formal high school at age thirteen, I received credits for only one year, since French was a high school requirement. I was able to take two years of French in one year since I could concentrate on this area because the other subjects were essentially a review of material I had already studied.

A board of three unpaid trustees, in most cases local farmers, supervised the one-room schools in the farming areas. The trustees had a number of responsibilities that included dismissal of teachers, which seldom happened, hiring a new teacher if a vacancy occurred, and auctioning various jobs necessary for the operation of the school. These included janitorial work such as the daily sweeping of the floors, oiling the wooden floors once yearly, and cleaning and polishing the stove used for heating the building as well as the stove pipes that ran the length of the building and were located about twelve feet above the floor. In cool weather the fire had to be lit early enough to warm the building for the start of classes. The school lawn of about one acre had to be cut once a year. A farm mower pulled by a team of horses did this. The least appealing job was cleaning the outside toilets, which consisted of two three-holers, one for the girls and one for the boys. The residue had to be buried near the privies.

The biggest job was the provision of firewood, which had to be cut a year in advance so that it would dry out for burning the following year. Chainsaws had not been invented; the trees had to be felled by a crosscut saw, powered by two men, one pulling on each end. Extreme care had to be taken when the trees were felled. Men have been killed by falling trees, which sometimes come down in an unexpected direction. After the tree was felled it was cut into blocks of wood short enough to be used as firewood and then split with axes into manageable pieces. Two persons on average could cut and split about one face cord of wood per day. A face cord is a pile of wood four feet high and eight feet long, with each stick about sixteen inches in length. In the winter the wood was drawn to the school by a team of horses pulling a farm sleigh. Seasoning of the wood, which took a year, occurred at the school.

Auctioning of these various jobs usually took place between Christmas and New Year's. The contracts were given to the lowest bidder, with the provision that if the work were unsatisfactory the individual would not be allowed to bid the following year. In my early teens, my brother Don and I obtained most of the contracts for the school, except for the janitorial contracts, which I could not do after I went to Dresden high school. However I continued to bid for, and usually got, other contracts, such as the ones for providing the firewood, cleaning the outhouses, and cutting the grass.

In 1932 my family purchased an additional 100-acre farm for two thousand dollars. My mother was very upset about the transaction since money was scarce. My father, as a carpenter, had a good knowledge of timber and saw it as a promising investment. He constructed a small building on the property to house employees and hired two local men to harvest the mature trees to be sold as logs. The men were paid the then going rate of one dollar per day per man. In addition we harvested firewood for the school from this farm.

Logging was normally done during the winter months, and the men finished the tree harvest during the second winter. We sold the logs, obtaining enough cash to pay for the farm. We have a picture taken in 1918, reproduced on the cover of this book, of a logging operation on the same farm.

Prior to our purchase, the farm had been owned by a Mr. Dalton who also owned a tile yard. This factory manufactured clay tile, used for the drainage of farmland. The timber from this property was burned in the tile kilns to supply the heat needed to cure the tile. In retrospect, huge amounts of hardwood timber must have been used for this purpose. At the time it was not realized that this was a waste of good timber.

In "The Story of Fairbank Oil," Patricia MacGee complains that "Most history books report, inaccurately, that Colonel Edwin Drake was the first to discover oil (in North America), at Titusville, Pennsylvania in 1858." She goes on to point out that "On August 28, 1857, the *Sarnia Observer* newspaper reported on the abundance of oil that the owners of the land were making available for lighting." (Source: Patricia MacGee, "The Story of Fairbank Oil," Browns Graphics and Printing, Inc., Petrolia, Ontario, 2004.)

Black Creek flows through our farm and empties in the St. Clair River. Upstream the creek passes through the village of Oil Springs. When oil was discovered in this area, some of the wells blew with so much pressure that they were called "gushers" and overflowed, flooding the creek with an oil slick to a depth of three feet. This oil eventually reached the St. Clair River. Perhaps the name of the creek evolved from the overflow of the black oil or from the tar residue along the stream and that led the early oilmen to the discovery of oil in the area. This bush lot is considered as a Carolinian property, since it has flora and fauna such as butternut trees normally found in properties of this nature. Efforts were made to transfer the land to the Nature Conservancy of Canada, which has an interest in preserving such unique properties.

Unfortunately this transaction could not be completed. My sister Margaret and I had inherited this farm after my mother's death. Two logging companies showed interest in acquiring the property. Had this happened it is probable that the property would have been clear-cut, and we did not want to see this happen. A young apprentice electrician who loves the outdoors and did not want to see all the beautiful trees harvested approached us. Eventually we agreed to a sale price and were pleased to have this young man become owner-custodian of the property.

Chapter Four

Growing Pains

During the war years, gasoline was rationed for most people operating motor vehicles. Since this fuel was necessary to operate farm tractors, farmers enjoyed a guarded exemption from the policy. Tractor gasoline had a dye added that turned the carburetor a blue colour so that an inspector could catch a culprit who used tractor gasoline to power his automobile. Demands for manpower in other areas was great, so inspectors were scarce. Predictably, few farmers observed the rule.

Uncle Blake operated a barbershop in Windsor. He and his wife Lillian frequently came to the farm to visit our family. It was not unusual for him to telephone my mother on a Sunday morning to invite himself and his wife for Sunday dinner. When his call came my mother would direct me (I would have been about eleven or twelve) to catch a chicken for the roasting pan. The chicken had to be decapitated, then eviscerated and plucked. On more than one occasion the devil in me suggested that one of the old cluckers mentioned earlier could be used.

What could be more fun than substituting a tough old hen for a tender young roasting chicken? It would be easy to say that simple good sense dissuaded me from such a prank; it is much more likely that I feared the wrath of Uncle Blake and my parents.

Uncle Blake always brought lots of candy for the kids. He brought his barber tools as well, to give free haircuts to all of the family. After the haircuts he often complained to my father that his gasoline was low, and could he "borrow" some of the tractor fuel? On one occasion, a snowy afternoon, the gas barrel for the tractor was empty. We had to siphon the fuel from the family Dodge. The siphon had been mislaid; I removed the plug from the bottom of the fuel tank of the car and caught the liquid in a pan. I poured the fuel into Uncle Blake's gas tank, but some of it accidentally spilled on my left sleeve. I went to the kitchen to wash up with hot water from a heating reservoir at one end of the wood stove. When the wash pan was full of warm water I decided, without thinking, to toss some wood pieces into the firebox of the stove. My sleeve passed over the open firebox. Gas fumes exploded!

I immediately ran out of the house and dived into a snowbank with my arm between the snow and my chest. The flames were quickly extinguished. Our local family doctor was able to apply a dressing, preventing infection and minimizing scar formation.

My only other experience with our family doctor concerned an athletic injury, a fractured clavicle (collarbone). I was about twelve at the time. What I remember most was the eighty-miles-per-hour ride in the doctor's car, over clay and gravel roads, to the Sarnia hospital. In the thrill of speed, I forgot the pain.

We had no electrical power on the farm until 1937. Up until that time we extracted drinking water from a drilled well. A windmill pumped water for the cattle to water tanks. We humans pumped our own drinking water by hand and carried it in pails into the house. In retrospect, when one considers the devastating effect of the recent outbreak of water-transmitted E. coli to the citizens of Walkerton, Ontario, the farmers of years gone by were most fortunate. In the year 2000 a virulent form of this bacteria seeped into the wells of the town from the manure of a local herd of cattle. Proper inspection and treatment of the town's water supply would have prevented this disaster. When one considers that the water wells for most farms were located in close proximity to the barnyards, it is amazing that outbreaks of E. coli toxicity were not more common in years gone by. Perhaps the farm people developed some immunity to the bacteria.

During the winter we had to break the ice on the water tanks used by the cattle so they could drink. During very cold weather the pump itself would freeze and had to be thawed by pouring in some hot water. I remember those days when I turn on a tap.

Children of today would be interested to know that water for personal hygiene was provided by rainwater directed from the roof by pipes draining to a concrete holding tank in the basement of the house. In many farm families baths normally took place on Saturday nights, whether or not they were necessary. Prior to electricity being available, we used outdoor toilets, very inconvenient if nature called on a stormy night! As a backup to the outdoor privy, we could use the chamber pots under the beds, but we had to empty them the next morning.

As a change from chicken, pork, and beef, our family enjoyed rabbit meat. My dad gave me a single shot 22-caliber rifle when I was eleven, as well as adding meticulous safety instruction for its use. Just before darkness of a day late in the fall of 1937, I was returning from a rabbit hunt. In the distance the recently installed electricity sprang to life. The house, barn, and other outbuildings lit up like something in a fairy tale! Half a mile away, I was sufficiently impressed to remember the sight to this day. Does anyone, in these early years of the third millennium, ever stop to marvel at the miracle of electric light?

The advent of electrical power was a wonderful assistance to life on a farm. We installed an indoor bathroom and included items, such as a toilet, bathtub, and washbasin, now considered commonplace. Hot water came from an electric tank as opposed to being heated by the wood stove. Incandescent bulbs replaced oil lamps and candles, improving our ability to study. Various electric motors and hand tools made indoor and outdoor work much easier.

The Great Depression of the 1930s brought disaster in many forms: financial crises, unemployment, loss of homes and jobs, and, in nature, terrible drought. One summer we had the lowest rainfall ever recorded. Crops all but ceased to exist. A ten-acre field of alfalfa produced only one-half a wagonload of hay, when during a normal year it should have produced twenty wagonloads. This hay was needed for the winter-feeding of cattle. Since there was no hope of having enough feed for the animals, we had to sell some on the open market, usually at a fraction of their real value.

Most of the world suffered during the depression years. In the United States, Franklin Delano Roosevelt, elected in 1932, opted for a large number of make-work programs to assist the unemployed. In Germany another new leader, Adolph Hitler, opted for another method of make-work for unemployed Germans. He commenced building a huge war machine and by so doing employed vast numbers of Germans in the hope of conquering the world.

During my formative years my father and mother relied on the good advice and assistance of the late Dr. Raymond Parr, a veterinarian who practised in the village of Brigden, about eight miles from the family farm. Many contemporary people would not realize the financial disaster facing a farmer during the depression years if a good cow or horse died from any cause, particularly from something preventable. Dr. Parr was greatly respected by his farmer clients. There is no doubt that my final decision to become a veterinarian was made easier by my admiration for Dr. Parr.

It is not always possible to help animal patients, as the following incident from the 1930s demonstrates. The local clay roads were maintained through the use of road scrapers pulled by a team of horses. A road scraper consisted of a flat steel platform on which the driver of the team stood to direct the horses. Beneath the steel platform were two sharp steel plates that stood on their edges, vertical to the steel platform. You might compare the scraper to a giant cheese-cutter skate. The blade smoothed the surface of the clay roads as the team pulled it. Something frightened the horses and they bolted; farmers call this a "runaway team." The driver was thrown from the road scraper, and the frightened horses galloped out of control. The bouncing scraper hit one of the horses above the hoof, severing the Achilles tendon. This beautiful horse had to be destroyed. Even today it is unlikely that a horse with such an injury could be saved, since this tendon is very large and heals very slowly. The size of the animal and the necessity to keep minimal weight on the affected leg while healing complicates the process.

My parents taught me many things, including the need to accept personal responsibility for my mistakes. I once found a dead female red fox, killed by an automobile. I could detect obvious signs that she had been nursing a litter. I searched for, and finally found, her den. One of the fox kits was still alive, so I decided to adopt the little creature. My father advised against the adoption of a wild animal as it was unlikely that it would become domesticated and in time it would revert to its wild heritage. I pleaded with him that this would be different, and eventually he allowed me to keep the animal. I nursed the little fellow with a rubber nipple on a milk bottle filled with cow's milk. It was normally used to feed orphan lambs. The fox kit always rapidly drained the bottle. As it increased in size, I fed it solid food, and the rapid growth continued. The fox kit, named Red, became as tame as a puppy and delighted in following the humans around the farm.

When Red got to be about six months old, he would wander away on his own. I should have known that my lack of supervision was a bad mistake. As a financial sideline, my mother raised turkeys. These birds were allowed to nest in the fields and raise their offspring without human assistance. In the late fall the turkey poults were almost full grown, ready to be sold. One day we heard a great commotion. Investigation showed that Red had killed all of the young turkeys. This was a substantial financial loss for an impoverished farm family.

My father took me to one side and told me that the fox had to be destroyed and that it was my duty to kill it. He reminded me that we had previously discussed accepting responsibility for our decisions. My mistake was my inability to take his advice that it is almost impossible to domesticate a wild animal. On many occasions during my years in veterinary practice, I have given the same advice to my clients.

Dad handed me his shotgun (much more humane for this purpose than my .22 rifle) and a shovel. I shed many tears as I buried the little fellow. I have never forgotten the lesson of accepting responsibility for my actions.

The reader will note that my regard for my parents was strong. My father used to smoke a pipe as well as cigarettes and, on special occasions, a cigar. My Uncle Blake, a frequent visitor to the farm, smoked one cigarette after another. Perhaps they were my role models. To be fair it should be stated that more than sixty years ago the hazards of smoking had yet to be understood. Even as an eleven- or twelve-year-old boy, I felt smoking seemed to be the thing to do. It was not too difficult to steal a few cigarettes and sneak out behind the barn for a few puffs.

One day they caught me. The sentence was to smoke my father's pipe, well used, loaded with the various obnoxious chemicals toxic to a little boy. After a substantial episode of vomiting, I was cured of the habit for a few days. Too bad it didn't last! If a reader of this discourse can accept a bit of advice, avoid addiction to nicotine!

In those years the men smoked in the house and went outside to go to the bathroom. How things change!

Draft horses provided the power to perform work now done by machines such as tractors. Three breeds of horses were the most common: Clydesdale, Percheron, and Belgian, big, gentle beasts. My father purchased a huge Belgian horse from a farmer who lived about twelve miles away. It was my job to ride him home. I was eleven years old, and my legs were not long enough to straddle his wide back. I had to ride bareback from the sidesaddle position. Several times I slid off the back of the horse, and since he was so tall I had to find and climb a fence to reach his back and resume the journey, a long, slow trip on a very patient animal.

We owned an old Percheron mare, which was afflicted with some intestinal disorder that resulted in loud gaseous explosions at frequent intervals. One day a neighbour boy and I decided to conduct an experiment on the characteristics of the gas. When ready to pass flatus, the old mare would lift her tail seconds before the explosion. My buddy and I lit a match at the precise time to determine whether the gas was flammable. It was! A streak of fire, at least a foot long, shot out! Luckily our prank did not result in a barn fire. We were badly frightened; the horse seemed unconcerned.

Hogs are different from horses in that they are temperamentally unpredictable. This is most noticeable in male hogs known as "boars." Boars develop elongated incisor teeth called "tusks." Adult boars are large animals, often weighing 500 pounds or more.

The father of one of my boyhood friends, Alex, kept a large boar in a pigpen. One afternoon when his parents were away, we decided to have a "boar hunt." Each of us had a BB gun that fired small lead pellets that would sting but not penetrate. After we had fired a few of these pellets at the boar through the window of his pen, he understandably became very annoyed. The angry animal jumped through the window of his enclosure and began to chase us. We ran to a woodpile, reaching safety just ahead of his chomping teeth. For what seemed to be several hours, the boar circled the woodpile, continuing to show his rage, trying to climb to our safe area. Had he been able to reach us, there would have been little doubt about our fate.

Alex's father came home and was able to chase the boar back to his pen. We received a well-deserved stern reprimand. A boyish prank had almost ended in the deaths of two thoughtless children.

Prior to our graduation as veterinarians, we were required to get field experience with practitioners. On one such occasion my preceptor and I were called to a farm to examine a cow that had been eviscerated. Our first thought was to check the barnyard area for a sharp projection that may have caught her abdomen, causing the wound. We were unable to find one. Suddenly we saw a large boar, which occupied the same barnyard as the cattle, and watched this big hog attempt to rip the abdomen of another cow with his tusks. The diagnosis became clear.

Every cattle farm needed a bull to fertilize the cows. Today the majority of cows conceive as the result of artificial insemination. The bull was normally kept in a pen until his service was needed, at which time he would be put with the cow. Most bulls had their noses pierced and a thick brass ring inserted through the penetration, allowing control of the animal by means of a hook that engaged the ring. Farmers on occasion became careless when handling the bull and sometimes did not live to regret their mistake. Because of his massive size, the bull would either crush the person or gore him with his horns if they had not been removed. As veterinarians we were very careful when we had to treat a mature bull.

Chapter Five

Dresden High School

The principal at the Dresden school agreed that I should repeat grade ten since I had taken no French at the one-room school. All of my new classmates were strangers.

My parents found a private home owned by a widow named Mrs. French, who agreed to provide me with room and board from Monday to Friday each week. It turned out that one of her sons, Glen, was to be a classmate, so this was helpful. Eventually he graduated from university as a civil engineer. Glen's older brother, Goldwin, graduated from a religious college and subsequently became a professor in Religion at an Ontario university. Mrs. French was a delightful person who became almost like another mother to me. Her two sons became surrogate brothers.

On Monday mornings my father would drive me about two miles to the home of the Evans family, who also owned a farm. Their daughter Wilhelmina was also a student at the high school but in a more advanced class. During the winter the concession roads were not ploughed. If the snow was too deep for a car to navigate the roads, my father would deliver me to the Evans's farm by horse and cutter and pick me up on Friday afternoon. One winter the roads were impassable for the whole season. I studied the rear end of the horse from the seat of the cutter twice weekly. Fortunately the country road in front of the Evans's farm was kept open all winter, or we all would have missed a school year.

I found the courses, except for the double workload in French, very easy. Mr. Stinson's instruction at the country school had been very helpful. Unfortunately, good grades came easily, and I became very bored with school. This attitude worsened with each year of study. During grade twelve I made the decision to leave school as soon as the year was completed. My parents, especially my mother, were devastated. They tried hard to persuade me to reconsider, without success. My father's advice was simple and straightforward; he said that it was obvious that I did not want to become a farmer, so I had to make a decision about my future. My sixteenth birthday had just passed; I figured I had plenty of time to think about that. It took several years for me to learn that my parents were right and I was wrong about leaving school.

Chapter Six

The Harvest Excursion

In the fall of 1942, advertisements in the local newspapers beckoned young men to Western Canada where farmers needed assistance in harvesting their crops. Grant Turner, son of a farmer who lived near our home, and I had been in the same classes throughout public school. We decided to join the harvest excursion. Ten dollars would take us from Sarnia, Ontario, to Westlock, Alberta, about fifty miles north of Edmonton, and home again. The train was slow and the tracks were rough. The seats were wooden with no cushions. The only food was sandwiches purchased from the conductor. The trip to Alberta took about four days. The hard seats and poor diet gave me a severe case of bleeding hemorrhoids, an affliction that corrected itself after the conclusion of the trip.

Jobs near Westlock had been prearranged. The farm where I was to be employed was about eight miles from town. The living quarters on this farm consisted of a combined kitchen and living room with an adjacent separate building for sleeping accommodations. There were four children in the family, the oldest a boy of about thirteen, the next a girl a year younger. Curtains separated the beds. It did not take me long to figure out what caused the bed springs in the parents' bedroom area to rattle so loudly!

My first job was to cut a large field of alfalfa hay. A mower, pulled by a team of horses, cut the stalks with a shuttling horizontal blade. These extremely sharp blades worked about two inches above the ground on the right side of the horses. Attention was required to cut along the line of standing hay to be sure that there was no obstruction such as a stone that would damage the blade.

Down one line, just in front of the blade, the standing hay appeared to move. Thinking that it might be an animal hiding in the long hay, I stopped the horses to investigate. I found brother and sister, naked in the grass! Perhaps the rattling bedsprings had instructed the children as well as the hired man!

Strong arms were needed to toss the sheaves of wheat on the horse-drawn wagons at harvest time. The fully loaded wagon was driven to a tractor-powered threshing machine in one of the fields. The sheaves were then forked into the threshing machine to separate the grain from the straw. It took several men with teams to keep the threshing machine in full operation. The harvest completed on one farm, the men, teams, and machinery moved to the next, where the procedure was repeated. As well as using the hired help, the farmers exchanged work with each other.

Harvest hours extended from daylight to dark. Such strenuous labour required large amounts of food. Breakfast was served about 5:30 a.m., sandwiches at 9:30 a.m., lunch at 12:00, sandwiches again at 3:30 p.m., and supper at dark after the horses were fed, watered, and brushed down.

We arrived one day to harvest a new farm. The kitchen, as well as what was visible in the rest of the house, was filthy. The odour of the place was almost unbearable. A baby in a carriage was covered with flies attracted, no doubt, by the smell of dirty diapers.

Our teams were tied to a fence between the house and the barn. An altercation broke out between two of the horses. One kicked the other so hard that a severe fracture occurred in one rear leg. The injured horse belonged to my friend Grant's team. The next day when we came in for lunch we saw the injured horse dead in the barnyard. A number of pigs crowded around the carcass, devouring it, but we noted that one rear quarter of the horse had been removed.

The reason for this soon became apparent. The farmer's wife announced that as a special treat she was serving roast beef for lunch.

As Grant cut his meat I heard him say, "Bess, I will miss you; you were a great horse."

Chapter Seven

Two Weeks in the Air Force

In 1942 the Second World War raged; German bombs pounded Britain.

While the minimal age for enlistment in the services was eighteen, many lads below that age signed up by falsifying their birth certificates. I decided that if some of my friends could join up this way, I would also give it a try.

The Air Force sent me to the Manning depot in Toronto for induction into the service. About two weeks later the officer in charge requested my presence. He told me that the forgery of my birth certificate was a lousy job but that if I wished they would like to see me in after my eighteenth birthday.

Chapter Eight

A Winter in Toronto

After my "discharge" from the Air Force, my mother's sister, Pearl, invited me to live with her family in Toronto for the winter. Since most of the able-bodied men were in the service, jobs were plentiful. I found work in the East Toronto steel fabricating plant of the Canadian National Railway. Railway bridges built at this plant were shipped all over Canada for installation. My job was to cut steel beams to a required length using an acetylene torch.

In the evenings my cousin Bob and I hung out together. One evening he introduced me to an acquaintance. An hour after the introduction this so-called friend drew a silver coloured pistol out of his pocket and suggested that we hold up a store. Finding his suggestion repulsive, we tried to think of a way to get out of the mess.

We took a bus some distance out of the city. The chap could not be talked out of his plan, so we left him on the bus and took another back to the city. At about 2:00 a.m. two policemen came to our door to inquire about the previous evening. Perhaps the boy with the pistol may have contacted them or someone else may have recognized us. The police must have been satisfied with our explanation; we were not contacted again.

A few days later I was working on top of a pile of steel girders some fifteen feet high when I heard a clatter in front of me. Suddenly a hand grasping a shiny pistol appeared over the pile of steel beams. A face, which I recognized, followed. I threw a steel wrench; it clattered across the beams.

The face disappeared. That was the last time that I ever saw that chap. Bob told me later that the so-called friend had been in jail for some crime. I have often thought how easy it would be for a boy to be talked into participating in a criminal activity without ever considering the consequences.

Chapter Nine

Steamboat Days

In March of 1944, after I had returned to the farm from Toronto, it was time to start a new venture. Sarnia, only twenty miles from home, was the logical choice to look for new employment. Most of my Toronto money had evaporated, so a new job was imperative. A newspaper advertised employment as stevedores loading freight on the package vessels that were plying the Great Lakes.

I applied. As in Toronto, there was a scarcity of labourers and acceptance was immediate. Paying a week's rent at a rooming house took almost all of my available capital. Two days of eating restaurant meals exhausted my funds. For the next three days I loaded heavy freight on the ships on an empty stomach. I had to eat, so I went to the boss to get a draw on my first paycheque; he was not sympathetic to my plight. I resigned, was paid off, and devoured my next meal in haste!

The port of Sarnia was home base for oil tankers that loaded at the local petroleum refineries and transported various types of oil products as far north as Fort William on Lake Superior and as far east as Quebec City on the St. Lawrence River. I applied to the Imperial Oil Company for a job on one of their tankers. Again, because of the shortage of labour, they took me on immediately. I joined the ship on March 29, 1944 (my eighteenth birthday), as a fireman.

A heavy-oil product known as "Bunker C" fired the ship's boiler. The oil flow of this product was fed to the boiler by a series of valves. The fireman's duty was to adjust these valves as necessary to keep the steam in the boiler at the proper pressure. When the ship was in port, minimal steam pressure was needed to keep the electrical generators operational and the hot water supply functional. When the ship began to move, adjustments were made to the valves as necessary. At full speed the valves needed little adjustment.

My first tanker, the Windsolite (name later changed to Imperial Windsor), sailed under the command of Captain Charles Dion, a real gentleman, strict when rules of his vessel were concerned but kind to his crew. He became a good friend. Many years later, after I graduated from veterinary college and started a practice in Scarborough, he telephoned me to say that he had retired and would like to see me again. During the early nineteen fifties, we spent many pleasant evenings with Captain Charlie and his wife.

The working day was divided into shifts: six hours on duty, then six hours off duty. These six-hour tours of duty were called "watches" and during a period of duty an employee was said to be "on watch." The six hours on watch with six hours off went on for seven days a week from the time that the ice broke up in the spring until the lakes froze again at the start of the next winter. Each ship needed approximately thirty men to operate efficiently. The crew included a captain who was completely in charge of all aspects of the ship. Duties were delegated to the following officers: under the captain was a deck crew of three officers: first mate, second mate, and third mate. Under the direction of the mates, the helmsmen steered the ship when it was in motion. Lowest on the totem pole were the deckhands, who did assorted jobs, such as keeping the ship clean and handling ropes (known as "lines") when the ship left or entered port. These lines tied the ship to the dock.

The engine-room crew was composed of a chief engineer as well as second, third, and fourth engineers. The engineers took responsibility for all mechanical elements on the vessel. Below the status of engineer were the oilers, who kept the many moving parts of the machinery lubricated. The final members of the engine room crew were the firemen, whose duties are described above.

Except for the officers, most of the crew were about my own age. The Second World War still raged, so most of the former Great Lake sailors had joined the merchant marines. Instead of plying the fresh water lakes, they sailed the oceans of the world, leaving a group of young, inexperienced men to replace them.

When teenage boys got together, then as now, there was lots of mischief. One of the boys adopted a small, black, stray mongrel pup as a mascot. The pup sailed the waters of the Great Lakes with us and seemed to enjoy himself. We stopped frequently at Toledo, Ohio, a short trip from Sarnia. Although we were all underage, we would visit a dockside tavern to enjoy a few beers. Our little mutt would accompany us to the bar. One of our guys would put some beer in a saucer, and the little dog rapidly developed a taste for it. Before long the regulars at the bar started to buy beer for the dog and for all of the dog's friends, as well. At the time I was not aware that dogs could enjoy alcohol so much. Later, in my practice, I treated several cases of severe alcoholic poisoning in dogs.

My duties on the tanker were a completely new experience and took a period of time to learn. It wasn't the first time that the engineers had trained a boy from the farm. More than once they warned me that an oil tanker, filled with fumes, could explode like a bomb. They insisted that rules be obeyed, particularly those related to safety.

I obeyed their advice without question.

Still, there were scary moments.

About 6:00 a.m. one morning, our ship prepared to enter the heavy ship traffic of the Detroit River. I had just come off watch from the engine room and went up to the deck to get some fresh air. We travelled "light," having just discharged our load of aviation gasoline in Toronto. For some time after unloading this fuel, tanks remain full of explosive fumes. A large white ship, an American passenger vessel, approached our portside much too close for comfort—probably less than fifty feet from us!

It would be safe to bet that none of the passengers on that vessel ever knew how closely the occupants of both ships approached oblivion. I would guess the captains of both ships shared equal responsibility for this near disaster.

One of the hazards of working on a ship is inclement weather. Our tanker took a cargo to Fort William (now Thunder Bay), the top of Lake Superior. We rode "light" (a nautical term for "empty"). A "light" ship rides high in the water and is much more susceptible to wind. On the return trip a few hours after we entered the lake, an unexpected storm blew up. The largest and deepest of the Great Lakes, Lake Superior can be wild; it has claimed many ships as victims. The elements battered us for hours. The waves were so large that the projections from the bridge of the ship (called the "wings of the bridge"), normally high above the water, dipped into the crests of the waves. To add to our discomfort, it was late in the sailing year and bitterly cold. The galley pitched so much that it was impossible for the cook to prepare fresh meals. We settled for cold beans. Dining tables on ships usually have rails along the edges to prevent dishes from sliding, but the plates slid around so madly that it was almost impossible to eat. Some of the men were violently seasick at the table. A disgusting mess of beans (eaten and uneaten) rolled erratically around the table! The storm raged for several hours. When it abated we were happy with the ability of our officers, who had steered us safely through.

The Great Lakes can be very treacherous during a storm. Lake Erie is relatively shallow, and when a strong wind blows, large waves soon arise. The rolling of the ship worsens when it rides sideways to the waves as opposed to heading directly into them. A short time after I had been promoted to Fourth Engineer, our vessel left the Welland Canal, bound west on a return trip to Sarnia. As we hit the open water, the wind strengthened and we headed directly into the waves. The ship pitched so much that when the bow rode a wave the stern would drop much deeper into the water than customary. This in turn would make the engine work much harder than usual, necessitating increase of steam power. When the bow then plunged into a trough, the opposite occurred; the propeller rose above its normal depth, so the engine would race to the point that there was the danger of it being thrown from the ship. When the engine raced in this manner, the throttle had to be adjusted lower to reduce speed. This changing of the speed of the engine lasted all of one night. During my shift I had to handle the throttle and adjust it as necessary. Because of the instability of the ship, it was necessary to hold the throttle with one hand and grasp a rigid support with the other. Again the crew appreciated that our officers had the knowledge and ability to get our ship through the crisis.

Chapter Ten

Change of Attitude

In 1946 I joined another vessel in the Imperial Oil fleet. By this time my mother and father had convinced me that I should consider returning to school. Four years had elapsed since I had made the regrettable decision that I had completed my formal education. It became obvious to me that while the pay on the ships was good and for a while this life was fun, there was little long-range future there for me.

This change of attitude was gradual and required a lot of soul searching. My parents, in particular my mother, were largely responsible for my changed priorities.

Mother knew that I enjoyed working with animals and knew of the great respect that I entertained for Dr. Parr, the caregiver for our farm critters. She contacted Dr. McNabb, Dean of the Ontario Veterinary College, to inquire whether I could be considered as a student. Dr. McNabb replied that if I completed grade thirteen with good grades, consideration would be given to my application. With a clear goal in life, and a new enthusiasm, I enrolled for my grade thirteen studies at the Petrolia high school early in 1946.

Bus transportation was then available for farm kids going to high school. Since I was now twenty years old, I was offered the responsibility of driving a small bus for the transportation of children in my area. I was elated with the position since it made a little extra money available.

The year at Petrolia High School was fun. As at Dresden four years earlier, I had no problem in achieving good grades, perhaps even more easily because of my changed philosophy. When the marks were submitted to the college they accepted my application.

College Years

Chapter Eleven

September, 1947

In September, 1947, my parents and I loaded the family car with my necessary belongings and drove to Guelph for the beginning of college. None of us had seen a college campus prior to that day. Formal registration was followed by a search for a place to live. I fell in behind a long line of students waiting to be assigned campus accommodations. There I struck up a conversation with the chap in front of me, Roly Armitage. We seemed to enjoy each other's company and decided to share residential facilities.

Slightly older than I, Roly had more than four years of overseas service as a war veteran. As I had done, he forged a birth certificate, but he didn't get caught. He had no high school training. At the end of the war the government of Canada set up a program of special rehabilitation schools where students could receive high school instruction from grade nine to grade thirteen in one year. Roly completed the entire five years of high school in one year—a monumental task.

Roly was from Carp, a small village near Ottawa. Soon after he returned from overseas he married Mary, his childhood sweetheart. Roly and I roomed together with two other veterinary students for the first year. Before the end of our first year, Mary told Roly that she was pregnant. The next year she moved to Guelph, where they found a small apartment near the college.

The colleges used several buildings on campus to provide accommodation for single students. The Ontario Veterinary College was combined with two other colleges, Ontario Agricultural College and the MacDonald Institute, to form what eventually became the University of Guelph. The Agricultural College offered a variety of courses related to this industry. The MacDonald Institute had two types of training for women. One offered a four-year course leading to a degree in home economics. The other, which the male students of the other two Colleges referred to as the "diamond ring" course, lasted only one year. It seemed to the egotistical males that the only reason for the one-year course was to provide the young ladies a happy matrimonial hunting ground.

Some of our professors were hard taskmasters with respect to workloads. Dr. Batt, Professor of Physiology, insisted that we learn every word on every page of his 500-page textbook. To navigate around this impossible task we reverted to making educated guesses as to what was likely to be on his examination.

Roly took Dr. Batt's advice and tried to memorize every lecture word for word as well as every assignment for homework. He asked me for help, and I told him that he had to pick and choose and commit to memory the most important material. It was fortunate that Roly learned to study properly, since after the Christmas examinations of our first year twenty-nine of our class failed to achieve a passing grade and were dropped from the student enrolment. We should have expected this culling of our class, as we had been warned in the early lectures by one of our professors, as follows: "Educating students is much like planting rows of carrots. One should plant too many so that when the gardener comes along he can pluck out one on either side of the strong and healthy carrot, allowing it more room to grow." He concluded in his droll manner, "Look on either side, gentlemen. After Christmas those seats may be vacant."

Dr. Victor Brown, who had the nickname of Tricky Vicky (behind his back, of course), was another who believed that hard work was good for students. He taught anatomy and insisted that the student remember the name and location of each bone, muscle, nerve, and each everything else that comprised the body of the animal. In addition we had to know the various structures and organs in a wide variety of animals.

The musculature as well as other anatomical structures around the head and neck of the horse is complex, so I decided to acquire a good learning aid. The head and neck of a horse became available. I took it to my room on the fourth floor of the dormitory. Fortunately there was a window with an outdoor balcony where I could keep my study specimen.

Dr. Frank Schofield was a pathologist who specialized in the study of the effect of various disease processes on the tissues of the body. His ability and outstanding research in a variety of areas were known all over the world. In 1923 he discovered that a fungus that grew on sweet clover was responsible for cattle bleeding to death following removal of their horns. This finding led to the utilization of coumadin, a drug still widely used in human medicine to assist in the prevention of clot formation.

After his retirement from the veterinary college, Dr. Schofield went to Korea, where he was instrumental in starting a new university that was quickly accepted as a fine institution. Before his death in 1970, Dr. Schofield received the highest civilian award from the president of Korea. The president, as well as the National Assembly speaker and some 900 other dignitaries, attended his funeral. More than 1000 mourners were at his graveside when his ashes were buried. Prime

Minister Chun delivered the eulogy to the man many Koreans called "Tiger Papa." Dr. Schofield is still known as the 34th man of Korea's independence movement.

In addition to being an outstanding pathologist, he was active in religious activities. Any student caught using alcoholic beverages was subject to severe criticism. A second conviction could lead to expulsion. On Sundays he would extend luncheon invitations to several student members. The purpose of these invitations was to interrogate the invitees on their attitudes regarding many aspects of life. Acceptance of these invitations, need I add, was obligatory.

A healthy rivalry arose between the students of the Ontario Veterinary College and the Ontario Agricultural College. This rivalry blossomed mainly in the area of intramural sports. Either group of students could dream up a sophisticated practical joke on the opponents. The first Halloween of our sojourn in college, a group of students stole an outdoor privy from a farm outside the city. They re-erected it that night at the top of the flight of steps that led to Creelmann Hall, the main student dining room. One student, after a heavy night of imbibing, decided to wait for the dining room to open. He believed, mistakenly, that this new building on the steps of Creelman was a rain shelter put up for student convenience in the event of inclement weather. He promptly fell asleep in this odoriferous accommodation, only to be awakened by the flash of a camera held by someone who wanted to get a once-in-a-lifetime photograph. Authorities conducted an intensive search for the culprits, but guilt never settled on anyone. Naturally the Aggies (Agriculture Students) blamed it on the Vets (Veterinary Students) and vice versa.

In 1947 the total enrolment of the three colleges was less than two thousand. The University of Toronto, with which the three colleges were affiliated, granted the degrees upon completion of the studies. Today as the University of Guelph it stands alone and has more than fifteen thousand students. In addition to the original three, a wide range of degrees is offered.

My mother's sister, Aunt Pearl, maintained, along with her family, a home in Guelph. Frequently she would ask me to join them for Sunday dinner. On one occasion I was reluctant to accept.

We had played a practical joke on a classmate, a chap known for his ability to sleep so deeply that anything could happen in his room without his knowledge. We mounted the body of a large, red, very dead rooster with strands of surgical wires, one under each wing and a third under his tail. During the night we attached the bird to the springs of the mattress on the bunk above the victim, the beak set about four inches above his nose. We put a raw egg in the toe of one of his slippers and then made so much noise outside his door that even he would awaken. This worked, and the big toe was immersed in raw egg. When he jumped to attention, the rooster "pecked" him on the nose!

He found the identity of the culprits and gave notice to expect a reprisal. That's why I was reluctant to visit Aunt Pearl.

But I did, and when I returned and unlocked the door to the room it jumped out of my hand. Suddenly I was soaking wet. The pins had been taken from the hinges and a large bucket of water had been delicately suspended by means of a rope so that when the door swung in the slack allowed the bucket to fall. There was not a single piece of furniture to be seen in the room. Even my desk and books were missing. All of the students pleaded ignorance, but one suggested that perhaps I needed to visit the bathroom after all of the excitement. Sure enough, all of my furniture was lined up in neat rows next to the urinals and toilets. One of my roommates had to be aware of this prank or the perpetrators could not have gained access to the room through the locked door.

No doubt the wide variety of practical jokes resulted from the need to relieve the pressure from the heavy workload we all shared.

Spring, 1948. Final examinations! A group of us decided to play a game of softball. I was the catcher for our team and had a foul tip strike the end of the right index finger. In addition to the severe discomfort, the digit lay terrifyingly at a right angle to the remainder of the finger—obviously a fracture. After X-rays a small cast was applied.

The invigilator in charge of the examination said, "Graham, if you think that you can escape writing this examination with the excuse of a cast on your finger, you can forget it." It had not been my intention to be excused, and I spent the next few days writing examinations with my thumb and second finger, with the index finger extended.

Chapter Twelve

Summer, 1948

Early in May students returned to their homes for the summer. Some of the Westerners discovered an arrangement that gave them a stipend and a free ride home. They would drive new cars from the factory back to Western Canada and deliver them to the purchasers. My mother heard about this arrangement and insisted that some of the boys stop at our farm for the first night on the road. This became something of a tradition. The regulars included Bob Green, Jack Greenway, Harold Hunter, Tom Sewell, and Larry Sparrow. Except for Harold and Larry, both of whom died at an early age, all of them are still great friends. It is my hope that prior to leaving this earth, Larry forgave us for his introduction to the red rooster.

A memorable regular of these year-end visits was Bob Green. He and my sister, Margaret, were married in 1951. I was asked to speak at the fiftieth anniversary of their marriage and wrote the following for the occasion:

Sow's Ear to Silk Purse

When I was a boy on the farm, my father taught me many things related to animals. One that I have not forgotten was his lecture about feeding stray cats. He discussed the importance of these critters in the control of rodents. He also said that since cats are very prolific and need food and accommodation, they would often arrive on one's doorstep with the hope of being looked after by some gullible human.

You may wonder what this dissertation has to do with a fiftieth anniversary wedding party. Let me explain: In 1947 a group of aspiring veterinarians registered for training at the Ontario Veterinary College. The students were seated alphabetically for lecture classes. Accordingly, Green and Graham were seated side by side. My parents suggested that I invite some of these students to have supper and spend the first night of their trip to the West. Bob, of course, was one of those included in the invitation. This became a yearly event. If I remember correctly, on the second year of this gathering of impoverished students, my sister Margaret had by some means received a respite from her nursing duties and was able to join the group for dinner. Veterinary students are trained in the art of diagnosis, so it did not take me long to deduce after the second or third annual visit of the students that there was a distinct possibility of a forthcoming romantic involvement. Margaret and Bob fell in love and were married fifty years ago. Unfortunately I was interning in California and was unable to afford the trip to attend their wedding.

Margaret and Bob have raised a wonderful family. Despite medical problems, they are hanging in and are a wonderful help to each other. There is an old saying that goes as follows: "Never feed a stray cat or you will have it for life." I would like to change this and say I am glad that my parents fed a few veterinary students.

Summer, 1948

*Please raise your glasses and drink a toast to their
fiftieth anniversary.*

Unfortunately Margaret was in hospital for treatment of
cardiac disease on the date scheduled for their anniversary celebration and has been in hospital off and on ever since. When
she is well enough to attend their postponed celebration, I will
be honoured to make this toast.

After exams I again went to work on one of the oil tankers
working out of Sarnia. This time, again because of the scarcity
of help, I was promoted to the post of Fourth Engineer, supervising the oiler and fireman on watch and directly responsible
to the Chief Engineer. The junior officers had better eating and
sleeping arrangements than the regular crew.

Later that year a seaman's strike resulted in the unionized
ships on the Great Lakes being tied to their docks. Since officers
were not unionized, we lived on the ships for the duration of the
strike, approximately two weeks. There was adequate food in the
stores, and we cooked for ourselves since the cooks were among
the strikers. Some of the strikers were quite militant. If we
wanted to go ashore, we went in groups for personal protection.

Another benefit of being a junior officer was a regular invitation to the poker games that the other officers played almost
every night. The stakes were relatively high for the time. With
good luck and some skill, my winnings kept increasing. From
time to time I would send some money to my mother for deposit
in a bank. I never told her the source of the funds—obviously!

Early one July morning, after an all night poker game, we
entered the St. Lawrence River en route to Montreal. The captain failed to avoid some rocks that were too close for the ship
to clear. We came to a grinding halt. Inspection revealed substantial damage to the hull. We limped to Montreal where we
had to be put in dry dock. It was estimated that repair would
take approximately two months. The chief engineer, one of the
big losers in the poker games, decided that a good job for me

would be repainting all of the areas above the boiler. The job appeared to be very extensive and would, without doubt, last for a good part of the repair time. The hot weather made the temperature over the boiler intolerable. It was my opinion that this onerous duty was directly related to my poker winnings. Accordingly, I handed the chief my resignation and took a train home. From May to July that year, wages and poker put two thousand dollars in my kick—enough to cover the expenses of my second year at college. I spent the rest of the summer helping my father with the harvest.

Second-year students were assigned better living quarters, and most of us lived with one roommate instead of three others as was the case in the first year. Fewer distractions made it easier to do homework.

The studies of the second year at college were similar to those of the first year. We still studied the basic material necessary to understand the complexity of diseases: anatomy, physiology, pathology, bacteriology, virology, parasitology, and so on. Eager to learn about the problems to be encountered in practice, we could hardly wait until the third year to study this material.

Agricultural economics, another of our studies, took the form of incredibly boring lectures delivered by an elderly gentleman. Most of us were unprepared for his final examination and would have failed except for the efforts of Bob Green, who had majored in this field at the University of Alberta prior to coming to Guelph. Bob patiently instructed us on the basics of this subject the night before the examination. As mentioned, Bob married my sister Margaret and has been a wonderful brother-in-law ever since.

Chapter Thirteen

Summer, 1949

After the second year of college, Bob Green, Joe Wellington—another classmate—and I drove to Nevada. A student a year ahead of us had worked the previous summer for Dr. W. E. Steinmetz, a Las Vegas veterinarian. Bill was highly recommended as a fine preceptor with an affinity for Canadian students. He agreed to take me as an intern and obtained positions for Bob and Joe with two of his colleagues in Reno.

Bob's old Jeep station wagon became our lifeboat of transportation. Throughways in 1949 existed only as dreams in the minds of planners, so the trip took almost a week on the two-lane highways networking the western states. When we arrived in Reno, their employers met Bob and Joe and me. After a short visit I took a bus to Las Vegas, a trip of close to ten hours.

Dr. Bill Steinmetz's clinic and his home were on the same lot at the north end of Las Vegas. His wife provided meals, but since their home was small I had to find accommodation in a nearby rooming house.

Dr. Bill was an excellent practitioner. He spent a lot of time instructing me on the art and science of veterinary medicine. His clients were impressed with his knowledge and ability as well as his empathy for the patients. I caught his enthusiasm for the work, deriving a spiritual energy for the next college year when we would start our formal instruction on animal diseases.

Soon after my arrival, Bill left to attend a veterinary conference. His wife, a graduate nurse, and I were left to look after the practice. At that stage of study I had almost no experience in the practical aspects of veterinary medicine. The day after he left, a cat hit by a car was admitted as an emergency. My first surgical procedure was about to take place! A few days earlier the same cat had undergone abdominal surgery in our clinic. Now the incision was ruptured and the intestines had eviscerated. Substantial contamination of the prolapsed organs had occurred as the result of being dragged through the dirt. Bill's wife, very cool and collected, directed me in the repair of the damage. The cat survived. It had used only one of its nine lives!

Las Vegas was at that time a boisterous community whose principal industry was gambling. The downtown area where most of the gambling establishments were located was so brilliantly illuminated that I was able to photograph night street scenes using the slow film speeds available at that time without flash bulbs. At the north end of the city lay an area that the locals called "the strip." At that time there were four hotels devoted essentially to gambling. Now an excess of fifty hotels on the strip exploit the industry.

The four opulent hotels did their best to make life comfortable for their guests. Each hotel tried to outdo the competition by featuring big stars from Hollywood. One could enjoy the entertainment provided by the famous performers for the price of a hamburger and a beer. Meals and drinks were very cheap, even for a student making twenty-five dollars per week, but you had to approach the restaurants via the gaming areas.

The town was built on a desert useless for farming since there was no rain to speak of. The desert, however, served my purposes in that it was easy to dig a hole in it. One of my jobs was to dispose of dead animals. After dark, when such disposition was necessary, I would take these corpses to a site north of the existing hotels on the strip and inter them. I have often thought that builders of the multitudes of new hotels must have uncovered my burial sites. They must have wondered about the origin of the bones!

Occasionally I visited the casinos. Short of funds, and conservative in nature, I wagered only minimal amounts. One evening I was shooting craps and bet one dollar at each roll of the dice. Each time I won I removed the dollar from the table, instead of letting it ride as most people might do. A large, smiling man was betting on me each time I rolled the dice. After twelve consecutive wins, I finally lost. The chap betting on me smiled and said, "Good rolling, kid," and tossed me a fifty-dollar chip, worth two weeks wages! He could afford it, since he had bet two hundred dollars each time I rolled the dice.

Las Vegas gamblers tend to be very superstitious. A lady client of our practice served drinks in one of the casinos. One morning she came in sporting a wide, elated smile. I asked about her good humour.

"I was serving cocktails last night to an elderly woman at the roulette table," she told me.

"I'm sure you do that every night."

"But last night she was tipping—believe it?—a hundred dollars each time she got a drink!"

"Impressive," I said.

"Sure is! I served her eighteen drinks! How she could stand up, let alone concentrate on the roulette wheel?"

Las Vegas had another industry. The state of Nevada permitted divorces provided that the person requesting the dissolution of marriage became a resident for thirty days. Most of the Las Vegas applicants came from Los Angeles. Reno was the preferred destination for applicants from San Francisco. People said that there were so many women in each of the above communities that houses of ill repute were unable to make a living due to free competition!

One of the potential divorcees from Los Angeles lived in a rooming house that happened to be my residence. She was a few years older than I and very attractive. Her new Lincoln convertible and impressive bank account added to the attraction. She loved dogs and cats and, since I was a veterinary student, seemed very interested in me. After a month or so she proposed marriage. I considered—but declined—the offer.

In early September I left Las Vegas and made the trip by bus to Reno to meet Bob Green and start our trip back to Canada. Bob's preceptor, Dr. Joe Key, had planned a farewell party for us. The party lasted until the wee hours of the morning—a mistake, since we started to drive about 8:00 a.m. Our friend Joe Wellington elected to go back by himself. Since Bob's home was in Alberta, we drove straight north through Oregon and Washington. To save money we drove all night, frequently changing drivers.

About 3:00 a.m. I felt the right front wheel engage the gravel at the edge of the road. I came to attention. To my right I could see the lights of a town some 2000 feet below. There was no guardrail at the edge of the road!

Bob's family made us welcome, and we spent a few pleasant days with them. Our next trip, Alberta to Guelph, was again non-stop except for fuel and food. We made it in twenty-four hours on the two-lane highways. Super highways stretched ahead of us—in years, not in miles.

Chapter Fourteen

The Third Year of College—A Day That Changed My Life

Our class had spent the first two years obtaining a solid background in the basic studies that would lead to an understanding of the various diseases affecting a variety of animals. We entered our third year with great excitement.

A few more of our classmates had married during the summer months and had moved from the bachelor quarters occupied by the rest of us. We residents still ate our meals in Creelman Hall. A small area at the south end of Creelman Hall, reserved for those members of the faculty who had their meals on campus, was off-limits to regular students.

A beautiful young lady sat down to lunch one day at the table reserved for the faculty. I couldn't help staring at her. She wore a white uniform with white stockings and shoes. A white nurse's cap crowned her. A classmate, recognizing my admiration, said, "I'll bet you a dollar that you can't get a date with her."

With no idea how to approach her, I accepted. There was a small infirmary on the first floor of the administration building for the treatment of minor problems that might afflict the students. Two nurses staffed the infirmary, one an elderly, abrupt lady who terrorized the students. Obviously the delightful young lady must be her new assistant. I decided that an old football injury to my left elbow should be examined immediately and followed the pretty nurse back to the infirmary.

Our lives hang on a variety of seemingly irrelevant threads! The older nurse had the afternoon off—how different would my life have been had it been otherwise? The young nurse examined the elbow and couldn't find anything wrong. At this point I had to confess and apologized. She had a good laugh and accepted my apology. When I asked her name, she replied, "Barbara Baldwin."

That day changed my life.

When circumstance permitted, I would haunt the dining area until Barbara finished her meal and walk back with her to the infirmary. After a week or so, she accepted my invitation to attend a movie. I collected the dollar from my friend, gave it to Barbara for a souvenir, and told her that it was the luckiest dollar I ever had. I have often wondered what happened to that dollar. Perhaps it was spent on sustenance during our hungry times!

Three other students and I took turns using an old Essex car we had bought for $100.00. Worn out tires presented only one of its variety of problems. On my first date with Barbara, we experienced a flat tire. Barbara named the vehicle "Athlete's Foot." The name stayed until the car ended in a scrapyard the following spring.

About a month after we met, Barbara asked if I would like to meet her parents, Walter and Eldora Baldwin, who lived in Cooksville, an hour's drive from Guelph. I accepted immediately. Walter enjoyed football, so Barbara invited him on a Saturday afternoon in late October to one of the college games. What they really wanted to see was what kind of a guy their lovely daughter was dating. I guess I passed the test, since we were invited to have dinner with them at their home the following Sunday.

Walter was employed by Ontario Hydro, in charge of a hydro substation in Cooksville. As manager he was entitled to the use of a company-owned home on the same property as the substation. As well as her parents, Eldora and Walter, one of Barbara's sisters was present. This sister, Fern, had an obvious physical defect in that her head was much smaller than normal. In addition, she had a speech impediment. Eldora told me that the measles virus she had suffered during the pregnancy caused these problems. By now I was sure that Barbara would become my wife, and I was worried that the problem might be a genetic defect rather than the explanation given to me. When I got back to the college, I spent a lot of time in the medical library studying the problem. The literature had a number of cases describing the affliction and satisfied me that what I had been told was likely to be accurate. I was very relieved to rule out a genetic defect as the cause of Fern's affliction. Barbara's parents looked after her needs until they were too old to continue with her care. Eventually they found a nursing home that was very caring for Fern's well-being. She resided there until she died in her late sixties.

Before my third year was completed, we knew we wanted to spend our lives together. I proposed marriage; Barbara accepted. We decided to wait until I graduated a year later to have the wedding.

An unwritten rule stated that members of the faculty were not supposed to hobnob with members of the student body—a rule we ignored. Congratulations on our engagement came from all sides—faculty, friends, and classmates.

Following my custom, I had my marks from the Christmas examinations sent to my mother and father. For the first time since I had entered college, my average was below 75 percent. Their response came quickly: "What happened?" When I told them that a lot of my study time had been redirected to the courting of a wonderful young lady, they understood and asked to meet her as soon as possible. When my parents met my future wife, they were delighted.

In the meantime I found that I had a competition problem. Barbara had a male friend whom she had gone out with from time to time. Since we were enjoying each other's company so much, she told him about me and broke off with him. She let him down easily by introducing him to one of her best friends, Bunty Dillon. They eventually married, and in later years after Barbara and I were married we saw each other from time to time. Bunty Dillon was invited to be Barbara's maid of honour.

Chapter Fifteen

Summer, 1950

Veterinary students were required to spend two months in a meat packing plant and two months with a rural veterinary practitioner to get some experience in both areas. All meat in licensed plants must be inspected both before and after slaughter to ensure that it is safe for human consumption. Most meat consumers are not aware of the important role that the veterinary profession plays in ensuring that the meat is free from diseases that can be transmitted from animals to humans. Graduate veterinarians, assisted by trained laymen, do the inspection.

I was posted to Stratford, Ontario, from the middle of May until the middle of July, 1950. At that time a widespread epidemic of bovine tuberculosis infected the cattle population of Ontario. Compulsory testing of cattle eradicated it. Affected animals had to be slaughtered. Cattle testing positive, called "reactors," were sent to a slaughterhouse. There, inspection took place both before and after slaughter. If the disease process was very minimal, the animals were passed for human consumption. Most of the animals had widespread lesions of tuberculosis and were condemned. The carcasses ended up as fertilizer after sterilization at high temperatures. It was sad to see the destruction of large herds of purebred cattle. One farmer lost his whole herd of Angus cattle, some fifty animals, to this disease. Some government compensation, well below market value for the loss of the animals, was paid to the farmers.

After Stratford I spent the rest of the summer in Brigden, Ontario. My preceptor was Dr. Raymond Parr, for whom, as discussed earlier, I had a good deal of respect. As was the custom in those years—and is no longer permissible—Dr. Parr left for a holiday soon after I arrived, leaving his student to run the practice. Since I had to make farm calls, I needed an automobile. I bought a 1929 Model A Ford coupe. This car differed from "Athlete's Foot" in that I could rely on it.

In addition to tuberculosis, brucellosis, another infectious disease of cattle, could infect humans. This disease, responsible for spontaneous abortion in cattle, may be transmitted to humans by consumption of non-pasteurized milk from the diseased cows as well as by direct exposure to the bacteria. When a cow aborts, she often retains the placenta in her uterus. Manual removal is usually required. In 1950, plastic or rubber sleeves had not yet been invented. The veterinarian had to insert his bare arm—in a large cow, up to the shoulder—into the uterus and pull the placenta out. Exposure by this means resulted in a high incidence of the disease in veterinarians. In humans the disease is better known as "Undulant Fever." It has a variety of symptoms, including waves of high temperature followed in waves by normal body temperature; hence the name. The patient may experience waves of euphoria and depression, leading to severe mental disorders. Body rashes are common. Years after the initial disease, severe arthritis and/or heart disease may occur.

In the late 1940s the government sponsored a program designed to control brucellosis in cattle. It provided vaccination of calves, done by veterinarians, against the disease. Adult cattle were blood-tested to confirm or deny infection. While working as a student, I was called to a farm, located about five miles from our office, to vaccinate a group of fifteen calves. The vaccination completed, I returned to the office.

The telephone rang soon after my return. It was from the farmer whose herd I had just left. Several of the calves were extremely ill and seemed to be in severe respiratory distress. It took only a few minutes to return to the farm, where I found three of the calves dead and half of the remainder with severe respiratory difficulty. It was not difficult to establish the diagnosis of anaphylactic shock. Since this is what I suspected, I had an ample supply of adrenalin in my bag. I administered the adrenalin intravenously, and they quickly responded. Laboratory testing of samples from the tissues of the dead calves confirmed the diagnosis. Blood samples were taken from the mothers of the calves. All were positive for the disease. Pathologists postulated that the cows had transmitted an allergy to the disease to their offspring, and when the vaccine was administered the severe reaction resulted.

The incident weighed heavily on me. During our final year we were asked to document histories on unusual cases. I chose these findings since few similar cases had been reported in veterinary literature.

I was called to examine a sick cow. The cow couldn't even get up. The farmer who owned her and a group of local farmers assisting with the harvest stood around to watch my examination.

Very ill at ease, I listened to the heart. The abnormal sounds reminded me of something that had come up in one of our lectures the previous season.

"Well?"

I was on stage—front and centre. And it was my turn to speak.

"She may have swallowed a nail or a piece of wire that got into her food," I muttered. "It's called 'hardware disease.'"

"Hardware? A disease?" laughed one of the onlookers.

But the owner was serious. "What I need to know," he said evenly, "is will she live?"

I shook my head. "From the sounds, I don't think so," I said. "If we had caught it earlier...might have been able to take it out. But it sounds like it's got to her heart." I was going to say a little more, but the farmer had turned and was ambling heavily towards his pickup truck.

In a moment he was back, shotgun in hand.

"A healthy cow is worth good money," he snarled. "But sick or dyin' ain't worth..." He punctuated his sentence with a blast to the animal's head, killing her instantly.

He did not put down the gun but held it dangling in his right hand. "Open her up, Doc," he drawled. "Show me the wire."

Uneasily, I began to cut. The farmers watched silently. There! A piece of heavy fence wire about a foot long, embedded in the heart, had caused a massive infection. Confidence washed over me then like a Lake Superior wave. "Fluid accumulation," I said, drawing my knife around in a circle just above the heart.

The unsmiling farmer nodded. "I know your dad," he said evenly. "I'm going to call him up now and tell him you done good."

In most respects the experience I acquired during the summer of 1950 gave me confidence for being on my own in the beginning and later with the instruction from Dr. Parr. I saw a variety of cases. With the help of textbooks brought from college, I could study the cases in depth at the end of the workday. When summer ended I was ready for the final year of study and for the renewal of the courtship of my wife-to-be.

Barbara was constantly on my mind. I wrote every day, expressing my love and telling her that I could hardly wait until our marriage became a reality. And each day a letter came from her expressing the same feelings. Since it was almost 200 miles from Cooksville to Brigden and since we both had jobs, we were able to see each other only once that summer.

Chapter Sixteen

The Senior Year

Full of enthusiasm, the class of 1951 began the final year. Students talked about the experiences of the past summer as well as post-graduation plans. Some had already made arrangements to join established practices, while others had found spots to open new practices. I was still undecided and kept all options open. One of my professors asked me to consider doing further studies in pharmacology, leading to a master's degree in this field. The studies for this degree would be done at the University of Toronto. Interested, I applied for a scholarship and was accepted on condition of achieving adequate marks in my final examinations.

Barbara and I renewed our romance. We had a wonderful winter and spring. Because of my commitment to good grades, we resolved that I should concentrate on achieving a scholarship. Accordingly, we dated three or four times weekly as opposed to almost every day as we had the previous year. We set our wedding day for May 23, 1951, the day after graduation. Barbara, her mother, and sister made all the arrangements.

Often we would double date with some of my friends and their ladies. A classmate, and still a close friend, Jack Greenway frequently dated a girl named Ada, often with Barbara and me. The previous summer Jack had worked in British Columbia and enjoyed the company of a young lady while in that province. He had invited her to come to Guelph the following February to the formal dance, an annual student black-tie affair called the Conversat. Jack apparently forgot that he had extended this invitation and also invited Ada. When the lady from the west arrived and phoned him from her hotel, Jack was in big trouble! A group of us decided that the only thing to do was to help him cover. We decided that he would bring one of the ladies and leave her at one of our tables, then slip out and get the other and deposit her at another table with some more of his friends. Jack placed his two ladies strategically at opposite ends of the room. When it came time to dance, he would take one lady to the floor, finish the dance with her, and go back to dance with the other lady. When Jack was away his buddies would talk to or dance with the neglected lady. Our own dates knew about his scheme and did not divulge the facts. This went on for the entire evening, and to this day we believe that the ploy was successful.

We devoted the final year to the wide variety of problems requiring the services of our profession. The months passed quickly, and soon it was time for the final examinations. All of our class passed the finals. To the joy of my parents, I achieved adequate marks for the scholarship. My proudest moment, however, was the fact that my pal Roly Armitage also achieved first-class honours, a remarkable achievement considering that he had taken all of high school in one year at rehabilitation school.

In the spring of 1951, I became quite ill with fever, rashes, and general muscular discomfort. Between the college physician and the bacteriology laboratory of the veterinary college, brucellosis (Undulant Fever) was diagnosed. I had contracted the disease from one of the cows treated for retained placenta. A course of antibiotics eradicated the symptoms.

Since brucellosis can lead to a wide variety of long-range human health problems, I decided to abandon a career of treating farm animals, opting instead for specializing in the care of companion animals.

Early in 1951 I had a letter from Dr. Bill Steinmetz, my Las Vegas preceptor. Bill wanted me to join him in Sacramento, California. He had sold his Las Vegas practice in order to return to his home state. He asked me to assist in his new practice and told me that it was much larger and busier than the other. I updated him on our upcoming marriage as well as on the possibility of a post-graduate degree. He said that he would be elated to have us even if it was only for a few months.

Barbara and I discussed this opportunity and decided to accept, even if we were there for a short time. Our arrival in Sacramento was set for early June.

Dr. Gordon Boylan asked me to help with his practice in Dresden during the two-week interval between the completion of the final examinations and the issuance of degrees. His brother Harold had been a classmate of mine during my high school days there. Harold graduated as a lawyer a few years before I graduated, since he had not taken a four-year hiatus between high school and university. I had known Gordon when I lived in Dresden and welcomed the opportunity to help him. Gordon had purchased a new Studebaker as his practice vehicle, and I was the first to drive it.

My first country call with the new car was to a farm east of the village. Returning, I caught up to a farm tractor pulling a wagonload of hay. A deep drainage ditch filled with water was located on right-hand side of the road. Beyond the tractor, an automobile approached. I slammed on the brakes. The pedal went to the floor—complete failure! Three alternatives become apparent: hit the back of the wagon; drive into the ditch; or try to pass. I pushed the accelerator to the floor and zipped around the wagon. The driver of the oncoming vehicle must have thought I was out of my mind!

At the dealership the mechanic found a fracture in the master brake cylinder that had allowed the brake fluid to escape.

Gordon's wife Alma, the receptionist for the practice, took the phone calls, made appointments, and in general managed the office efficiently. One day while I was on a country call, she contacted me by radio to inquire about a dead dog that had been brought in by the owner for disposal. She asked me what the owner should be charged. "Charge him plenty," I replied, "the ground is hard and I'll have to dig the hole." What I didn't know was that the client was still in the office and had heard my intemperate remark on the two-way radio. Every time I see the Boylans, they remind me of the incident.

I had arranged to purchase a used Plymouth from a cousin who lived in Cleveland, Ohio. Just before graduation I flew to Cleveland to pick up the car and drive it back to Guelph. Since this car was to be our transportation to California, I decided to have new tires installed in the States before entering Canada.

The graduation exercise took place May 22, 1951, in bright sunshine, on one of the expansive lawns of the college. It was a proud day for the students, their wives, and wives-to-be, as well as their relatives.

My parents had booked accommodation at the Royal Hotel in Guelph for the night preceding graduation. When my father checked out, the desk manager handed him some of my baggage that had been stored at the hotel, since I had made reservations there for the night of my marriage to Barbara. Dad recognized my luggage and to his credit didn't tell a soul until he took me to one side after the wedding. He got a good laugh from my attempt to have a little secret.

Barbara's sister Evelyn Knott and her husband Steve had made arrangements for a stag party to be held at their home in Port Credit the night before the wedding. Invitees included her father, as well as some of his friends, my father, and a few of my classmates. It was a pleasant evening with limited amounts of alcohol. As mentioned earlier, my father had two beers, breaking his longstanding rule about consumption. The evening ended early in anticipation of the next day.

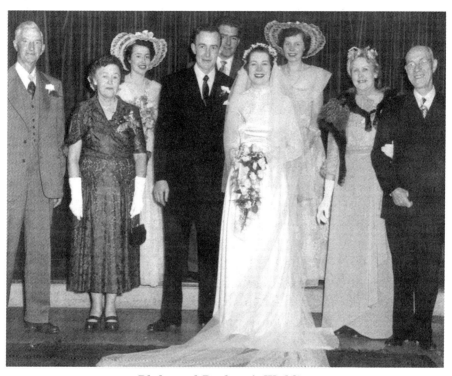

Blake and Barbara's Wedding
Left to Right: Edward Graham, Mary Graham, Margaret Graham,
Blake Graham, Roly Armitage, Barbara Graham, Bunty Dillon,
Eldora Baldwin, Walter Baldwin

The weather gods were with us again. Our wedding took place at Cooksville United Church in the early afternoon of a warm and sunny May 23. The bride was, as always, a beautiful lady, and I felt most honoured that she was soon to be my wife. Her long-standing friend Bunty Dillon was the maid of honour, and my good friend Roly Armitage was my best man. Following the ceremony a reception was held at a local restaurant. After the meal we returned to the Baldwin's home for more wedding pictures and a cocktail party in their garden.

Barbara and I returned to Guelph to spend our wedding night at the Royal Hotel and claimed our luggage. I told her about my father's little secret, and we both appreciated his discretion in not divulging where we would be on our wedding night.

The next evening we invited some of my classmates who had not left the campus to be our guests at another reception. We opened a bar in one of the dormitories for the celebration. Unfortunately one of our former professors came along and said that we would have to leave, since the party was against college rules. We knew this, of course, but had decided to ignore it. The party adjourned to the hotel and was enjoyed by all.

The following day we started our long trip to California. The first major stop was Chicago. We had been invited to visit the home of my cousin George Graham, whose father, David, was one of my father's older brothers. George and his wife Lillian were wonderful hosts. George was a graduate engineer with several inventions to his credit. One was a conveyor belt system designed to feed coal to the furnaces of big manufacturing plants. Another of his patents was a television aerial developed when television was in its infancy.

The next morning George invited me to go for a drive with him to see the result of another of his ideas. He had started a chain of self-service laundromats in various areas of Chicago. The coins from the machines were dumped into canvas bags and taken to a bank, where they were weighed rather than counted. George then suggested to me that if I would go back to Toronto and start a similar chain in that city, he would provide the necessary start-up capital. He assured me that this venture would be much more lucrative than working as a veterinarian. I had no doubt that he was correct in his assumption but did not want to waste the hard work of the past years.

We continued our way west. In Denver a large parade in progress brought the traffic to a standstill. To escape the jam,

I drove the car over a curb. At the foot of the mountains, a lunch stop was in order. As is my custom wherever I stop, I walked around the car to inspect the tires. I found a bulge on one tire. Part of the red inner tube protruded. Obviously the wall of the tire had been damaged when it had hit the curb. Since the tire was not safe, especially on mountain roads, I changed it and the journey continued. Eventually we found a dealer of that brand and replaced the damaged tire.

Our slow journey continued over the two-lane highways to Salt Lake City. The weather forecast for the next day—hot. We retired early so that our trip would start at daylight. The Salt Lake desert can be, and usually is, very hot in early June. This day was no exception, and we had an uneventful trip because of our early departure.

SECTION THREE

Veterinary Practice

Chapter Seventeen

The Sacramento, California, Veterinary Clinic

Dr. Bill Steinmetz and his wife welcomed us to Sacramento. He had rented a small apartment close to his clinic. This was to be our first matrimonial home. Shortly after our arrival, Bill and his wife left to attend a veterinary convention. As well as being responsible for the operation of his veterinary clinic, we had the job of babysitting their two children—an instant family after two weeks of marital bliss!

In those years each veterinary practice looked after its own emergencies. Bill's practice had facilities for nearly one hundred animals and most of the time operated close to capacity.

Shortly after I took over, a midnight emergency presented itself. I was running a high fever, caused by a large abscess on my backside. This may have been the result of my infection with brucellosis, exacerbated by the long trip in the car. I sure did not feel up to seeing the patient but had no choice. After Bill returned from the convention, we alternated for the provision of after-hours emergency service.

Barbara was offered, and accepted, a position as office nurse for a medical doctor in the area. It was a job she really enjoyed, since her employer was competent with the care of his patients and kind with his staff. Her working hours allowed us to spend most evenings together.

When we made the decision to work in the United States, we knew we would have to get a green card from the U.S. embassy. We did this in the winter of 1950–1951. A few months after our arrival, I received notification from the U.S. Draft Board asking me to report to San Francisco for a medical examination. This could lead to my induction into the U.S. service. The Korean conflict was raging, and I had no desire to become a participant. After a military physician examined me, I was informed that I had a pylenidal cyst (a cyst that is connected to the spinal cord at the lower part of the spine). He suggested that after I had and paid for the surgical repair, the service would accept me. I knew that his diagnosis was incorrect in that he was looking at the drainage point of the abscess. Notification came that I was unfit for service. Good news!

California requires a valid licence to practise, as do other states and provinces. To obtain such a licence one must obtain passing marks in examinations set by the jurisdiction. I decided to write the examinations for the state of California in late 1951. They were held in San Francisco and lasted for three days. The exams were very difficult, especially for someone who had been out of college for a long period of time and decided to practise in the state. It was easier for a candidate such as myself who had just completed college. There were many difficult questions, such as "Describe the udder of a cow." To answer this question properly, the examiner required that the candidate explore every detail of the subject. This included the anatomy of the organ, including the hair covering the skin, the skin itself, its blood supply, naming the arteries and veins as well as their anatomical locations, and the naming of the nerves, including their locations. In addition, the examiner wanted a description of the milk-producing glands, both from their gross and microscopic appearance. A description of the various ailments affecting the organ was required. To answer this question properly required about three hours. The three days I spent writing such difficult examinations were the most mentally trying of any three days that I had ever experienced. It was a great relief when the letter came stating that my licence was granted.

My association with Bill was of great benefit to me. He instructed me in many areas of companion-animal medicine new to me. When I made a mistake he was gentle with criticism, with the one requirement being that the same mistake not be made again. I really enjoyed being a practising veterinarian.

I notified the University of Toronto that I wanted to become a veterinary clinician as opposed to following research in pharmacology. They replied, asking me to reconsider, but my decision was final.

Our first Christmas as a married couple was a very happy one. We took a few days away from work to visit several areas of the state, including Sutter's Mill where gold had been discovered in 1849. Being deeply in love we delighted in having a few days by ourselves. We did not miss emergency calls in the middle of the night! We had lots of time to discuss our future. Bill had asked me to consider becoming a partner in his practice—a very inviting offer. Barbara was becoming a little homesick, since she had never been away from her family and friends for an extended period. I understood her concerns. We elected to defer any decision for a few months.

In January of 1952 we were happy to receive a letter from Barbara's father saying that he was coming to visit us. During his stay we discussed Barbara's concerns, a lot of which had to do with raising a family so far away from our roots. We told Walter that we would consider returning to Canada. He stayed with us for ten days and then took the long trip back by bus.

We both wanted to start a family but agreed to postpone decisions until our future became more clarified. We fully understood that our financial situation would have to improve prior to taking such an important step.

An interesting facet of Bill's practice was a contract to look after the health of the animals in the local zoo, a small operation displaying a wide variety of animals, including members of the feline species as well as various herbivores. One day the zookeeper brought a carrying case filled with lion kittens to our clinic. The reception room was full of dogs. It was amazing to see German shepherds and Dobermans, terrified by the odour of lion kittens, trying to hide behind their owners.

In addition to a variety of big cats, the zoo had a selection of primates and herbivores. These animals suffered a variety of problems that were a challenge to treat. We had regular visiting days at the zoo to monitor the health of our patients and to advise the keepers on preventative medicine.

The Sacramento Bee, a city newspaper, owned a large parrot that had lived in the offices of the paper for some seventy years. One day the bird was brought to our office with acute respiratory distress. Obviously it was suffering from a severe pneumonia. Penicillin was very new in veterinary medicine, and we decided that if there was any hope of saving the bird it should be administered. The penicillin of those years was combined with procaine, a local anaesthetic, to relieve the discomfort of the injection. An hour or so after the injection, the parrot expired. The newspaper published an account of the death in the next edition and was very complimentary about the care we had given. Several years after the incident, I read an article in one of our professional publications that noted certain experimental evidence had concluded that procaine was contraindicated in parrots. In all probability the praise for our services was not justified.

A client of ours owned a beautiful Irish setter whose name was Peter Chris Patrick the Third, nicknamed Pete. Pete had been trained as a bird dog, specializing in pheasant hunting. The owner was moving into a smaller home and could not keep him. Pete had a draining abscess on his left rib cage, and the owner requested that he be destroyed. I asked him if, rather than kill the animal, he would consider giving him to me. He readily agreed. Exploring the abscess, I found a small stick embedded in the wound. I removed this foreign body, and recovery was uneventful.

Rice is a common crop in California, and clumps of it provide cover for pheasants. One afternoon I decided to see whether or not Pete was the dog I thought him to be and could live up to his reputation as a bird dog. He came on a point near a small rice paddy, perhaps three feet in diameter. Seeing no evidence of a bird, I started to walk away. Pete looked at me as if I were stupid, then dived into the clump, emerging with a large male pheasant. Was I the person he thought me to be? Apparently not! The bird had a broken wing and was unable to fly. This did not preclude the enjoyment of a fine dinner. Pete came back to Canada with us and remained our canine friend for the next decade.

Barbara and I had many discussions about staying in California. It became evident that we would prefer to return to Canada and start a veterinary practice, probably in Toronto. I discussed our decision with Dr. Bill. He was disappointed but understood our position.

About the middle of February, we packed the Plymouth with all of our worldly belongings, which didn't even fill the car, put Pete on the back seat on top of the assorted goods, and started our homeward journey. We had an uneventful trip until the arrival at Port Huron, Michigan, in preparation for entry to Canada, well after midnight. The customs inspector stopped us to inspect the vehicle. When his head came through the window of the rear seat, he startled the dog that had been asleep and was greeted with a vicious snarl. We were waived through with no further questions.

Chapter Eighteen

The Danforth Veterinary Hospital

The village of Cooksville, home of Barbara's parents, stands a few miles west of Toronto. Walter and Eldora welcomed us and invited us to stay until we could find a practice location. By locating the various existing veterinary practices on a map, we were able to find a spot where no such service was available. At the east end of Toronto in the area of Scarborough, no practices devoted to companion-animal medicine existed. When we drove around the area, we became certain it would be a good location for my practice. We looked at several buildings in the area that were for sale, including an old butcher shop. The owner, retiring, was anxious to sell. He agreed on a price of $18,000.00 and offered to take back a first mortgage for half of the purchase price. My in-laws loaned us the money for the down payment, and the transaction was quickly completed. The property was situated at the corner of Danforth Avenue and Danforth Road. The name "Danforth Veterinary Hospital" seemed evident.

The Danforth Veterinary Hospital

The building consisted of a ground floor that could easily be converted into a clinic, a basement for storage, a one-bedroom apartment on the second floor, as well as a living room, kitchen, and bathroom.

We had little capital. After the expense of my college education, I still had a debt of approximately $2000.00. When my father heard about the purchase, he offered to come to Toronto and help with the necessary renovations. He was a carpenter and had the skills to make the necessary renovations. The changes were completed by mid April, and we opened for business.

Soon after we opened, two disconcerting events arose. A friend of the former owner came in as a new client and told me that the former owner was ready to foreclose on the mortgage as soon as I was unable to make the payments. I was determined to avoid this eventuality. A few days later I found that another veterinarian had bought a building on the opposite corner, planning to open a practice there. While my research had indicated that the area badly needed veterinary service, I was unsure whether two new practices could survive. The local municipal authorities notified me that they were reluctant to allow two practices on the same corner, citing traffic congestion as their reason. I hired a lawyer to deal with the municipal authorities. He succeeded in overcoming their objections. It turned out that the mayor of Scarborough was a buddy of the father of the veterinarian who had purchased on the same corner. While competitors in the beginning, my colleague Dr. Len Burch and I became close friends and often helped each other with difficult cases. Both practices flourished, since there were so many people in the area wanting veterinary service.

There was little money to furnish the apartment as well as purchase the equipment and pharmaceuticals necessary for the operation of the practice. Our dining table consisted of a sheet of plywood supported by two suitcases of uneven height. As a young married couple, we joked about our impecunious state. We could joke about it because we knew it would improve. Our bedroom was sited directly over the kennel room. Often at night we would be awakened by barking dogs; usually when one dog started the rest would join in. Worse than the noise of barking dogs was the odour of tomcat urine. Entire cats (cats that have not been castrated) produce a urine foul to the olfactory sense of humans but attractive to female cats and a deterrent to other males. Deterrent, indeed! When this odour infused the building, including the bedroom upstairs, there could be no doubt as to the source.

Barbara acted as office manager as well as surgical assistant. Pete, still with us, usually stayed at the top of the stairs and would come down periodically where the work was in progress, no doubt to measure competition for the affection of his owners. On one occasion a large green parrot was brought in for treatment. It stayed for a few days on the first floor and from time to time would whistle shrilly, bringing the dog downstairs to see who had called him. The parrot seemed to enjoy the game, and the dog never realized that he was being conned.

By the standards of today, fees for veterinary services in 1952 were modest. For example, the fee for an ovariohysterectomy— commonly known as spaying—of an immature dog was $7.50. Certain non-professional work, such as clipping and bathing animals, came to the clinics since there were no local establishments to provide grooming services. It required about an hour to clip and bathe a cocker spaniel, a breed quite popular during that era. Until my professional practice grew, we provided this non-professional service for the clients. Frequently I groomed five or six dogs a day to help cover the overhead expenses.

By the fall of 1952 the practice had matured enough to require the assistance of an animal attendant, who took over the duties of grooming, exercising the dogs, cleaning kennels, washing the floors, et cetera.

In those days injections were made with glass syringes of various sizes (as opposed to the plastic disposable syringes in use today). The glass syringes and the needles had to be washed and sterilized after each use. These syringes cost $2.00 or more each, depending on size. My new animal attendant sterilized about fifty of them one afternoon. While attempting to take them from the hot autoclave, he dropped the tray and broke every one—a financial disaster!

As the practice had grown very rapidly, Barbara and I decided that we could now reasonably consider starting our family. We discontinued birth-control measures. Very soon we were elated to learn that she was pregnant. Our respective parents shared our happiness. When Barbara had graduated as a nurse from Wellesley Hospital in central Toronto, she had developed a fondness and great respect for the professional ability of an obstetrician from that hospital, Dr. Tait. He agreed to supervise the pregnancy and made regular house calls. He liked to discuss comparative medicine with me, particularly about cases related to reproductive diseases. On one occasion, just before he arrived, I had completed the removal of a badly infected uterus from a tiny chihuahua. I kept the organ for his inspection, and he was amazed that the uterus with the contained purulent material was more than 25 percent of the weight of the dog. Apparently this condition, known as pyometra, while common in dogs is very rare in humans.

A client came in with a female red Doberman. He introduced himself as a dog trainer, recently arrived from Hollywood. He hoped to develop a facility dedicated to the training of guard dogs and believed that the Toronto area would be a good place for the new business. The Doberman did not appear to be aggressive and sat quietly during our discussion. I asked him the reason for training the Doberman. The trainer stated that the owner was a local businessman (whose name I recognized) and that this individual enjoyed relationships with other men's wives. He feared retribution and had purchased the animal for protection.

The trainer offered to demonstrate the dog's ability. The animal was wearing a choke chain attached to a leash. He asked me to stand a few feet from the dog and sharply jerked the leash. Immediately the dog lunged at my throat. He then gave me the leash and the process was repeated with the target being the trainer. The same thing happened. Jerking the leash was the dog's signal to attack.

I inquired as to his fee for training the animal and was told $2000.00. This seemed a huge amount of money compared to my office consultation fee of $2.00. There should be a way to add a few zeros to my fee structure! I never found out whether or not the owner of the Doberman received his money's worth. Or needed the dog's services!

Soon after the practice began, I received a telephone call from a magistrate who, in addition to performing his judicial duties, served as director of the local racetrack. This man invited me to attend his office to discuss a business matter. Intrigued with the thought of improving my cash flow, I met him. He offered to pay me $50.00 for two hours work per day to inspect racehorses to determine whether or not they were fit to compete. I told this gentleman that my knowledge of racehorses was very limited and that I could not be of much help. He replied that my limited knowledge was the reason for the offer and that my legitimacy as a veterinarian to sign the documents was all that was required. The inspections were to be done by lay people. Uncomfortable with such an unethical offer, I declined.

A veterinarian sees much of the pathos of human life. An elderly lady often came to the office with her pet canary in its cage. Invariably she would state that the bird had been poisoned. On her first visit she told me that she lived with her daughter and son-in-law. She would accuse the son-in-law of poisoning the bird. The canary always seemed perfectly healthy, so I tried to dissuade her from her fears. The advice would serve temporarily; a week or so later, she would return with the same problem. Without her knowledge I phoned her daughter, who knew about her concerns but was unable to rationalize with her mother. She suggested I phone the family physician. He told me that he was aware of the accusations and that always after her visit to my office she seemed better able to cope with her concerns. The visits went on for several months. Eventually the canary, quite old for a bird, was found dead in its cage at their home. Again the lady arrived with the bird and requested an autopsy. Although I told her that this would be a waste of money, she insisted. The examination, which included sending samples to a laboratory for toxicology, was negative as anticipated. She insisted on having the body of the bird returned. Several months later she sent me a letter stating that a taxidermist had stuffed the bird. She went on to say that it was still happily ensconced in its cage and was now safe from further attempts on its life.

Another elderly lady, a cat fancier, always dressed in the styles of the Victorian era. She told me that she was a teacher, specializing in dramatic theatre. She had an assortment of cats, one of which was very emaciated. X-rays of the abdomen revealed complete calcification of the wall of the aorta from the heart to where the artery split into the femoral arteries that descend to the rear legs. I told her there was no treatment for the condition. She took the cat home. A month or so later she arrived again, this time with a small wooden box containing the body of the cat. She told me that it was unconscious and asked if I could give it a stimulant to awaken it. A moment's examination showed that the cat had been dead for several days. Convinced about its state, she also made the decision to have a taxidermist preserve it.

A mixed-breed male dog fifteen years of age was presented for diagnosis of a large mass at the base of its tail. The mass was a large hernia known as a perineal hernia. This problem is related to lack of testosterone in aging dogs and results in the loss of the supporting tissue adjacent to the rectum. This allows some of the intestines to migrate and be contained only by the skin. While it is possible to repair the problem surgically, the owner must be informed that it is a long and somewhat dangerous procedure on an aged animal. After due consideration the owners made the decision to attempt the surgery and brought the dog back on a Saturday for the necessary pre-operation care, with the surgery to take place Monday morning.

The intestinal contents had to be evacuated in preparation for the surgery. I took the patient to a vacant lot next door for the evacuation. Because the dog was old, very friendly, and quite feeble, I did not think it necessary to put him on a leash. He completed his business of the moment. Suddenly, much to my surprise, he started to run, I in hot pursuit. At that time I was young and healthy and felt that it would be no problem to catch him. The dog was going in the direction of his home, and since he could run faster than the young veterinarian, I ran back for the car to continue the pursuit. I caught up to him as he arrived at the front door of his address. When the owners came to the door, I explained the situation to them and we all had a laugh at my expense. With a heart powerful enough to beat a young man in a race, it did not surprise me that he came through the surgery with no problems.

In the early1950s, prior to the discovery of rabies in southern Ontario, people often brought in young skunks they had found and wanted to keep. I told them that wild animals as a general rule do not make good pets, but many did not take the advice and requested that the sacs containing the powerful aroma be removed. This is not a very difficult procedure when the skunk is six or eight weeks old. It is somewhat harder when the animal is several months old.

A classmate of mine, Dr. Jim Lennox, had opened a practice in Weston, at the northwest edge of Toronto. He knew that I had descented a number of skunks and asked me to demonstrate the procedure. He arrived one evening after office hours with two skunks, one seven or eight weeks old and the other somewhat older. The smaller animal was anaesthetized with ether, and the procedure was completed with no problem. The same anaesthesia was used on the larger animal, and I removed one of the sacs. Jim then asked if he could do the second and proceeded with the surgery. Suddenly the room was enveloped with skunk perfume—he had nicked the scent bag! For those who have never experienced the aroma of a skunk, it can be overpowering. Jim had always been known for playing practical jokes, and I have always suspected, in spite of his denials, that this was not a surgical accident. It took several weeks for the odour to disappear from my building. This was the last skunk to have this surgical procedure done in my practice. We will never know the truth of Jim's story, since he died from a generalized malignancy.

In early 1953 I purchased a used X-ray unit—a major expense, but very often necessary for good diagnosis. While I was apprenticing in California, we admitted a dachshund with a gunshot wound. X-rays determined that the bullet had lodged between two of the vertebrae. Since this piece of lead could migrate into the spinal canal, I decided to operate. I utilized a foot-operated fluoroscope during the long procedure in order to keep the bullet located. Several months later my fingernails developed superficial cracks that still persist after fifty years. The problem, in all probability, is related to radiation from the long exposure to the fluoroscope. Several old-time veterinarians have suffered much worse damage, and some of them have lost parts of their fingers due to radiation from X-ray machines. One of our lecturers in college, a human radiologist, lost all sensation in his fingers from repeated exposure. To pick up a pencil he would have to look at it and at the same time close his fingers. After such a warning, and mindful of the evidence of my own fingernails, I was more careful with my new machine.

An old-time veterinarian, Dr. Vivian Banks, had a practice about five miles from ours. He had a large number of clients who bred English bulldogs. Because of their large heads and small pelvic girdles, most were unable to have a normal birth and required a caesarean section for delivery. He would ask either Dr. Burch or me, usually alternating between us, to assist with his sections. After I purchased my X-ray equipment, other veterinarians would, on occasion, bring their patients to my office for radiology. One such veterinarian was a classmate, Dr. Dick Ketchell, who later became my partner. One evening Dick brought in a young animal with severe pain in both elbows and unable to put any weight on either front leg. I took the films. While they were being developed Dr. Banks dropped in for a visit. Dick asked him for his opinion as to the cause of problem. He ran his fingers over the elbows of the animal and announced, "This dog has osteogenic sarcoma (a highly malignant type of bone cancer) with spontaneous fractures in both elbows." By now the films were ready and proved him to be correct. Dr. Banks at that time was more than seventy years old. He sure impressed us with his diagnostic ability.

By early August of 1953, Barbara was very pregnant and most uncomfortable because of the hot summer. Dr. Tait thought that she was overdue but did not feel it necessary to induce her. He said, "Give her time, and she will be fine." She still insisted on helping me with what had become a busy practice. The veterinary profession from Toronto and area, known as the Toronto Academy of Veterinary Medicine (TAVM), provided free professional service at the Canadian National Exhibition, starting mid-August and ending on the Labour Day weekend. My duty was for the afternoon of August 22. I tried to find someone to take my stint, but no one would. When I got back that evening Barbara had fielded the drop-in clients and was exhausted. An hour or so later she knew that she had to go to the hospital. In the early hours of August 23, our wonderful daughter Janet was born.

After a few days we were able to bring our baby home. Fortunately Barbara had spent a lot of time with babies while she was training to be a nurse and was well aware of what procedures were necessary to raise the infant. She began breastfeeding so that the maternal antibodies could be transferred to Janet. She was an easy baby to raise and, except for some minor episodes of colic, had no problems. Our dog Pete, in the beginning, seemed to be jealous of the baby but soon realized that he still had a place in the family and as time went on became very fond of Janet.

After about six months we decided that our living space was cramped and began the search for a new home. In 1954 we bought a new home on Sylvan Avenue on Scarborough Bluffs overlooking Lake Ontario. Our hard work and long hours spent building the practice had paid off. The mortgage on the hospital had been discharged (much to the surprise of the former owner), and we had paid off the loan from Barbara's parents. They offered to help finance the new home.

One of our clients, an English couple named Ed and Sylvia Harris with a young son, David, mentioned that the home that they were renting was no longer available and they would have to move. I suggested that they take over our apartment, rent free, for providing after-hours supervision. Happy with the offer, they moved in. Sylvia replaced Barbara and became a very competent salaried office manager. In a veterinary clinic it is important that someone reliable is available during the night for supervision of in-patients and for the fielding of after-hour telephone calls. Many of these are not true emergencies. If they couldn't make a decision as to whether or not the animal had to be seen, the call was referred to me. If the call was an emergency, such as a caesarean, help was required.

An example of a non-emergency phone call follows. Ed and Sylvia could not satisfy an inebriated woman who phoned in the middle of one night. When I called to find out about her concerns, she told me that there was a large spider crawling around her living room floor. I explained to her that there were no poisonous spiders in Canada and that she was in no danger. Not satisfied, she wanted me to make a house call and destroy the creature. When I refused this request, she became quite belligerent. I told her to put on a shoe and step on the spider. Before she could answer, I hung up the phone. It took a long time to get back to sleep after listening to such nonsense!

In those years vaccination programs against distemper, a widespread infectious disease of dogs, were unreliable. Three injections at two-week intervals were administered, resulting in some immunity for several months. Since it had been established that the immunity was relatively short, it was decided that after the three injections the dogs should be exposed to other dogs on the street or taken for walks in parks to augment any immunity derived from the vaccinations. This seemed to reinforce the immunity.

Since distemper was a virus disease, there was no effective treatment. The virus was capable of infecting any organ, including the respiratory tract, the intestinal tract, and the brain. Often three or four weeks after the initial symptoms of coughing, eye discharge, or diarrhea, the animal would develop nervous symptoms, which could include severe convulsions or muscular spasms. When these symptoms occurred, the result was usually fatal. It was a very disappointing to have a case presented with the initial symptoms since the owner had to be advised that brain damage often followed the initial problem. Because of better vaccines this disease, like polio in humans, is seldom seen by today's veterinarians. This does not indicate stopping vaccination programs, since there may be reservoirs of the disease in other parts of the world that could be spread to North America, resulting in the same devastating problem we saw fifty years ago.

I employed a part-time worker, Gladwin Watson, for general duties on Saturdays. He was about twenty-four years old. After he had been with us for a year, we decided to take a week's holiday and found a locum veterinarian to look after the practice. When we returned I phoned the locum to see if there were any problems and was told that our employee was in hospital with an unknown disease. I phoned his attending physician, who informed me that the lad was critically ill but no diagnosis had been established. We discussed his symptoms: vomiting, severe pain in his lower back, abnormal urine, and high fever. The physician informed me that Glad's parents were told the prognosis was grave. In California I had seen several dogs with similar symptoms, caused by a disease called leptospirosis. The causative organism is spread in urine of infected dogs and is transmissible to humans. The physician agreed that laboratory work should be done to eliminate or confirm the diagnosis. When it was established that the young man in fact had leptospirosis, he became a medical curiosity in the hospital since it was their first diagnosed case. Fortunately penicillin and streptomycin were available, and following the use of these antibiotics the young man made an uneventful recovery. I postulated that he had mopped up urine in the clinic from a carrier of the disease and without washing his hands had eaten his lunch. While I never saw a case of leptospirosis in my Canadian practice, it is probable that carriers exist in Canada.

I lost contact with Gladwin (Glad) until 2003 when he left a message on our answering machine without using his first name. Imagine my surprise when I returned the call and was connected to my friend Glad! A few weeks later he came to our cottage for a visit. I was anxious to see whether or not he had any chronic problems resulting from leptospirosis. Dogs frequently have chronic kidney or liver disease as an aftermath of the acute infection. Glad assured me that he did not have any such aftermath. He mentioned that he had to retire prematurely from his position with the provincial government. He was struck on the head by a piece of wood that had bounced off a truck. He gradually recovered from this unfortunate accident. We had a good visit and rehashed old memories.

Soon after opening the Danforth Veterinary Hospital, I joined the Toronto Academy of Veterinary Medicine (TAVM), whose members included most of the practising veterinarians in the general Toronto area. At that time there were two main goals in this organization: to provide emergency service to clients on nights and weekends on a rotating basis and to get to know each other as colleagues rather than as competitors. At that time there were less than thirty practising veterinarians in the entire area.

One Sunday while I was on emergency duty for the city, a Dalmatian dog was presented, with a severe laceration to one of its footpads. The owner had tried to control the severe bleeding with a bandage, but the wound required deep sutures to arrest the blood flow. It turned out that the owner was the American consul for Canada. He and his wife were charming people. They lived several miles from my office. They didn't have a regular veterinarian and asked to become my clients, to which, of course, I agreed. After a couple of years he was posted elsewhere and offered to sell me his automobile, a Buick sedan. He had purchased the vehicle at a discount since no duty was payable because of his position, and the purchase price was very attractive.

During my membership in the TAVM, I suggested that the organization consider regular meetings devoted to continuing education that would enable us to keep up to date. This idea was accepted, and we started to have monthly meetings with good speakers on a variety of subjects. The idea has persisted through the years and has been a great success for the interested practitioners.

In 1955 I was elected president of the TAVM. The position would last for a year. During my tenure the first cases of rabies in Ontario were detected. In my college years rabies was referred to as "Artic Fox Disease" and at that time existed only in the far north. Since as practitioners none of us had ever seen a case of rabies, the Board of Directors of the TAVM felt that we must upgrade our knowledge of it. We were all well aware that the disease in both animals and man is invariably fatal once the symptoms are manifested.

We contacted a laboratory in Pearl River, New York, where vaccines against rabies, for both animals and man, were produced. The head of the laboratory was most obliging and invited any interested veterinarian from our group to attend an information seminar. Most of the practitioners from our area decided to go, each paying his own expenses. Films were shown depicting various manifestations of the disease in animals and man. I will never forget the image of a man strapped to a bed in terminal convulsions as the result of the rabies virus.

We returned by airplane and arrived in Toronto about midnight. We hadn't been notified that a television crew awaited our arrival. Television was in its infancy, and none of us had ever seen a TV camera. The onus fell on me, as president of the group, to present our findings. The interview was aired the following day. Viewers were interested and we were asked to do another program on the same subject a few days later at a CBC studio in Toronto.

Because television viewers had shown a lot of interest in subjects related to pet animals, television studios requested that the TAVM participate in several other programs related to pets. Our association agreed, and this series was appreciated by the viewers who saw the programs.

Since rabies had not been a problem in Ontario, the supply of vaccine was limited. The only dogs vaccinated up until that time were those going to the United States or to other countries where the problem existed. To purchase even one vaccine, a veterinarian had to apply to the Health of Animals Division of the Department of Agriculture in Ottawa. When it became obvious that Ontario had the problem, vaccination against the disease was recommended and supplies of the product became available to private practitioners as well as to federal veterinarians. The animal-owning public wanted to protect itself as well as the animals, so widespread vaccination against the disease became routine. Since the major vectors of the disease are different species of wild animals, it is unlikely that rabies will ever be completely eradicated.

There are two forms of the disease: dumb rabies and furious rabies. An animal with dumb rabies becomes passive. Usually the lower jaw drops because of paralysis of the jaw. The furious form of the disease is frightening to see. The animal will attack anything. Cases have been documented where rabid foxes would attack railway tracks and break their teeth on the metal rails. A fox or skunk with the disease would attack a much larger animal, such as a cow or horse, in which case their saliva would penetrate the skin and infect the other animal.

One Saturday morning an owner brought a large chow for examination. This dog had licked one of its rear legs so hard that the skin was abraded. It was black fly season and the dog had been at the owner's cottage. I assumed that it had been bitten by a black fly and the animal's skin was irritated. I applied a dressing and dispensed a sedative. That evening, while dining with some friends, I received an emergency call. The owner said the animal was acting strangely and seemed aggressive. I suggested that the animal be restrained with two leads and that it be brought to my office as soon as possible. The dog was ferocious and had large amounts of saliva hanging from its mouth. No doubt we had a classic case of furious rabies. The owner and his son assisted me in confining the dog in a secure cage. I had to tell them that the animal would soon be dead; in fact, it lasted only a few hours. Fortunately they had not administered any of the oral sedative. I asked them if they or any of the rest of the family had been exposed to the saliva of the animal. They felt that no exposure had taken place.

Laboratory examination of the brain tested positive. I contacted their family physician, who had to make the final decision as to whether or not prophylactic measures were indicated for the family. He decided against such measures since the owners believed no exposure to saliva had occurred. It is likely that the dog was exposed to rabies at the owner's cottage. It had not been vaccinated against the disease and had free access to the bush around the premises.

By late 1955 the Danforth practice had grown so rapidly that the size of the building limited further expansion. The long hours and stress exhausted me mentally and physically.

Frequently my classmate Dick Ketchell and his wife Irene would visit with Barbara and me, either at their place in Port Credit or at our home in Scarborough. Dick's problems were similar to mine. The possibility of partnership in building a new state-of-the-art veterinary hospital frequently came up. I admired Dick's professional ability and was aware that he had been one of the top students in our class. We began to look for a suitable location for the new premises. I had a client whose job was finding new locations for a large chain of supermarkets. This company did extensive market research on population growth prior to purchasing a new property for one of their stores. We believed that the criteria used by this company would supply the same benefit for our purposes. They had chosen a new location at the corner of Markham Road and Eglinton Avenue in Scarborough. Directly across the street from the supermarket property lay a vacant lot. We made an offer for this property. It was accepted.

In early 1956 we employed an architect to design the building. Most architects knew nothing of the special needs of a veterinary hospital and required a lot of input from us as well as from available literature with respect to building plans. We submitted plans for bids and chose a contractor. Construction began in late 1956. Since so much of my time was devoted to planning and supervision of the construction of the new building, I needed a veterinarian to assist in the operation of the Danforth Veterinary Hospital. Fortunately I found a young graduate looking for employment, Dr. Ken Gadd. Ken was (and still is) an outstanding veterinarian. He married his beloved Margaret soon after he joined my practice, and Barbara and I were invited to the wedding. We had an extra bedroom in our home, so they lived with us for a few months. Ken and I shared the night and weekend emergency calls. This was the help I needed.

The American Animal Hospital Association (AAHA) is dedicated to the improvement of quality companion-animal treatment. The premises of a practice wishing to join this organization must meet strict physical criteria. Other requirements exist: proper patient records, adequate professional libraries, up-to-date equipment, and, above all, continuing education of the owners. It was our intention to qualify for membership in this organization.

We instructed our architect to obtain building plans from the AAHA and utilize them in planning our building. We had the completed building inspected to assure compliance with standards. Membership requires periodic inspection of the premises and of the professional practice to ensure that high standards continued. If a client were to move to another city in Canada or the USA and asked to be referred to another veterinarian, we could assure them that if they went to an AAHA member they could be assured of quality and fair service. During our years as members Dick and I rotated attendance at their annual conference, usually held in an American city.

Chapter Nineteen

The Amherst Veterinary Hospital

Telephone exchanges of 1957 had names instead of numbers. The exchange in our area was "Amherst," a name we felt would be easy for our clients to remember. We selected it as the name for our new institution. We needed two successive telephone numbers and were allocated Am 3322 and Am 3323, which became 261-3322 and 261-3323—again easy numbers to remember.

The new building was completed and ready for occupancy in May of 1957. Complications arose. It was not only the equipment and inventory that had to be moved; the hospitalized animals had to be transferred as well. We moved on a Sunday in order to make things less complicated for the clients. A few weeks ahead of time we sent letters to my clients advising them of the date of the opening. Notification was sent to various others, such as our distributors. The mortgage on the hospital was provided by a client who had expressed interest in the financing after becoming aware of the new venture.

Shortly before the building was completed, I received a letter from my friend and mentor Dr. Bill Steinmetz. Bill said:

Well, I am really pleased that your project is almost finished. Usually unexpected cost overruns will exceed your planned budget. Accordingly, how much do you need? Let me know by return letter, and I will send you a check.

He was right—our costs were approximately $10,000.00 over budget. I replied, and a cheque quickly arrived to cover the shortfall. His generosity has always been appreciated. We repaid him with interest.

Invitees to our opening included all of my clients as well as all veterinarians in the Toronto area. Dick and I acted as guides to show off the new establishment. Compliments abounded. All, including members of our profession, stated that they had never seen a more modern or efficient veterinary establishment.

Our euphoria was short-lived. The gates for the kennels were made of aluminum. We had contacted an American company that specialized in constructing animal kennels. When the architects saw the price of the kennel gates, they advised us that gates of similar quality could be manufactured in Canada for half the cost. We took this advice and ordered the Canadian product. About three weeks after the opening, we found that large dogs would bite the bars of the kennel doors and twist them so much that they could escape. In a few more weeks, most of the doors were ruined. The problem was obvious—the aluminum had less tensile strength than the American product. We immediately ordered replacement doors from the States and had them installed. Since we had not paid for the Canadian doors, we informed the company that we did not intend to pay for the defective product. They replied that since our architect had established the specifications of the product, they were not to blame and would sue us if immediate payment were not received. We consulted a lawyer who felt that we had a good case and that it should go to trial. I suggested to the lawyer that the architectural firm should become part of the suit, since they had, in fact, specified the tensile strength. The lawyer said that the architect should be kept as a friendly, as opposed to hostile, witness. The judge ruled against us and ordered us to pay for the doors. Since we had not implicated the architect in the original suit, our lawyer told us that it was too late to sue the firm. So much for good professional advice, both legal and architectural!

On the lower floor the new hospital had a comfortable one-bedroom apartment. Sylvia and Ed Harris moved with us and lived in the apartment. Sylvia continued to be our receptionist. Their son David by now had aspirations to become a veterinarian, and as the years passed this became an eventuality.

I sold the old veterinary premises to a local physician who modified the building to use as his office. He became a good friend as well as our family doctor.

From the opening in May until September when Dick joined the new practice after having sold his Port Credit location, I operated the new facility by myself. We stayed open seven days a week. Office hours on weekdays ran from 8:00 a.m. to 7:00 p.m. and on Sundays from noon to 3:00 p.m. I was on call every night. Dick's arrival in September was a great relief. Barbara, Janet, and I took a week's holiday for rejuvenation and visited a resort north of the city.

Dick and I decided that the practice should give the best possible professional service with a fee structure set between the highest and the lowest offered in other practices. This policy proved successful, and the practice grew rapidly. The veterinarian on duty offered the last client of the day a guided tour of the hospital. We were able to show all of the facilities: examination rooms, library, X-ray room, surgery room, treatment room, laboratory, grooming room, isolation room, and various kennel rooms. Invariably the client would comment that the facilities exceeded what had been expected. Often people who had heard good comments from friends would ask for a tour.

About this time Dr. Banks, mentioned above, retired and sold his practice to two young graduates, Doctors Bill Dale and Bill Whittick. After a few years of veterinary practice, Doctor Dale enrolled in medical school. He became an outstanding obstetrician and gynecologist. One day a regular female client brought her pet into the clinic for routine treatment. This lady was a registered nurse. It was obvious that she was very pregnant, so I asked her who was looking after her. She said Dr. Dale, who at that time was head of obstetrics at Scarborough Centenary Hospital. I said to her, in a very concerned manner, "Did you know that he is a veterinarian?" When she recovered, I explained that that was his original profession prior to becoming a physician. She was very relieved and had a good laugh, no doubt very happy that Dr. Dale was a "real" doctor. Bill phoned me later, also amused.

Bill Whittick, a veterinarian of above-average ability, both diagnostic and surgical, became interested in orthopedic surgery and attained board certification in this field. While still in general practice, he wrote a textbook on this subject that was used in many veterinary colleges around the world and, I am told, is still found and consulted in the clinics of many contemporary veterinarians. Frequently, in the evenings, I went to his office to photograph the surgical procedures that were to be used as illustrations in his textbook. The production of this book was an amazing achievement for someone operating an active practice. Bill must have had incredible powers of concentration. His brother-in-law wrote to me:

I have vivid memories of Bill writing that book. He did not, as I would have, work at a large, officious desk guarded by silent walls and locked doors, but sat in an easy chair in the family room with a sort of loose clipboard, scribbling away while four young children fought, ran, played war and cowboys and Indians around him, wife screaming from the kitchen for the kids to behave and the husband to get ready for supper, and the brother-in-law (yours truly) arriving for a visit, coming in the door, asking if there was cold beer in the fridge. How that book ever got written!?

When his book was published, Barbara and I hosted a book publication party for Bill and his wife Lynn. They were asked to submit a guest list of colleagues and friends to be invited. Many attended to honour his achievement. Guests came from Canada and the United States, many having travelled long distances for the occasion.

On the day prior to the book publishing party, Barbara suffered extensive bleeding from her uterus. We had known that she had fibroids, but they had not been a real problem. I suggested that we call off the party, but she was adamant that, since the guests were coming from long distances, we continue with the plans. The day after the party, Dr. Bill Dale, who had been one of the guests, performed an emergency hysterectomy. She had an uneventful recovery. I cite this incident to underline her tenacity and desire that friends should come before personal problems.

Working together, Bill and I presented several seminars in Canada and the United States. We had accepted an invitation to put on a two-day seminar for the veterinary profession in Montreal. The program was to start at 1:00 p.m. Our flight from Toronto was to leave at 9:30 a.m. I was to pick him up at one of the intersections of the 401 highway. Prior to leaving home, I phoned to say that I was on my way. When I arrived at the appointed spot, there was no sign of him. I waited as long as possible and decided that there was no alternative but to catch the plane by myself so the seminar could start on time. He arrived later that afternoon. He had waited on the wrong side of the intersection and stood there for a long time in a heavy snowstorm. Lynn, his wife, phoned Barbara and intimated that I had played a terrible practical joke on her husband.

We were to return from Montreal two days later. I took an afternoon plane. Bill decided to take the evening plane since he wished to visit some relatives. Because of demand, the evening flight was divided into two sections, Bill on the first. The second section, leaving an hour later, crashed on takeoff and had no survivors. We were both fortunate; the husband of one of Barbara's classmates was on the second section.

After he left general practice in Toronto, Bill taught orthopedic surgery at three different veterinary colleges. Later he opened a referral orthopedic practice in Miami, Florida, where he and his wife Lynn lived until his death from heart failure. He is missed by his good friends, both inside and outside the veterinary profession.

Chapter Twenty

Unusual Cases

Because Dr. Ketchell and I had diverse areas of interest, the partnership succeeded. Dick enjoyed orthopedic surgery, treatment of bird diseases, and radiology. I found particular interest in feline problems, ophthalmology, and practice management. We both had an interest in internal medicine and enjoyed solving complex cases.

My interest in ophthalmology was recognized by colleagues and resulted in referrals of problem eye cases. One hot summer day, a lady and her chihuahua were referred for an eye consultation on the dog. She had driven for about fifty miles and did not have an air conditioner in her car. Her attire, appropriate for the day, consisted of a skimpy halter, short shorts, and sandals. The dog, still nervous after the long car ride, draped his head over one of the owner's shoulders and his rear feet anchored in her halter. In the examination room the dog started to struggle in her arms. The struggle resulted in the strap of the halter breaking, with complete exposure of her bosom. Immediately she said, "Please take the dog and stop staring at my fried eggs." I include this in unusual cases since it was the only such occurrence during my years of practice.

The windows of the reception room extended from floor to ceiling, offering a good view of the parking area. A new Thunderbird, red in colour, and the first one I had seen, came in and parked. A young lady and her massive boxer got out of the car and entered the hospital. As she was a new client, she went to the receptionist for the necessary paperwork. This completed, we entered the examination room. I lifted the dog and placed him on the stainless steel examination table. I inquired as to the reason for the visit, and she told me that he was dragging his seat on the ground so she suspected that he had worms. This problem is usually not worms but rather impaction of fluid in the anal glands—two small sacs located on either side of the anus. I discussed with her the probable need of being cleaned out from time to time to prevent infection.

The lady told me that the dog disliked veterinarians and would likely try to bite me. She held the dog by its collar while I was at its rear end to attend to the problem. As soon as I started the procedure, the dog spun on the slippery stainless steel table. His snapping jaws came so close to my fingers! I tried to grab him by the leg but, due to his swift movement, missed his leg and grabbed his scrotum instead. This worked very well, particularly when I, by reflex, twisted it. The attack quickly subsided, and the dog remained docile while I completed the procedure. The owner, not knowing how the dog had been subdued, said, "My! You have a good way with dogs."

I replied, " Most dogs know that I am not afraid of them and recognize that I am the boss."

This client came in from time to time for anal gland treatment, as well as for other problems. Sometimes other veterinarians in the practice saw the dog and always complained to me how nasty it was. I never disclosed my secret to them. Every time that I saw him, this dog was always placid with me.

I consider this case to be unusual in that it demonstrates that the dog remembered me as the scrotum twister.

Animals are often brought to veterinarians for the diagnosis and treatment of skin conditions. An itchy skin may be a simple problem, such as flea infestation, or may be more complex, such as allergy to plants or to food ingredients. A client owned two unrelated German shepherds, both of whom were so itchy that their skin were abraded from scratching. After eliminating several potential possibilities, I suspected that they had a form of mange, caused by a tiny parasite. In humans the disease is called scabies. I asked the owner whether she or anyone else living with the dogs had any skin trouble. She said she lived alone with her dogs. She also informed me that she had a rash on her chest that had been diagnosed by her employer, a dermatologist, as an allergy to her nylon brassiere. I asked whether there was any direct contact between the skin of the dogs to her affected area, to which she replied in the affirmative.

This history made me all the more determined to confirm my tentative diagnosis of scabies. To confirm the diagnosis it is necessary to do skin scrapings and examine them with the aid of a microscope. I did several scrapings on the first visit and was unable to demonstrate the parasite. Still convinced that I was right, I had the lady come back on several occasions for further examination. Eventually I found the parasite and had the owner look at it with the aid of the microscope. These mites, too small to be seen without magnification, burrow under the skin causing severe discomfort.

I suggested that she go back to her employer and ask him to perform similar skin tests on her affected area. He was able to confirm that she had the same problem as her dogs. After treatment, both the lady and her dogs recovered without incident.

Dick had an unbelievable memory. We had a very difficult case referred by another veterinarian. The symptoms did not fit the normal pattern. After due consideration Dick said that he remembered a similar problem that had been reported some ten years before in the *South African Journal of Veterinary Medicine*. He went to our library to find the article, and, sure enough, he found that our case was identical. The final diagnosis was confirmed by laboratory tests.

On another occasion we had a dog presented with a severe cough, difficulty in breathing, and severe weight loss. X-ray examination disclosed large numbers of rounded, calcified areas in both lungs. The dog had lived in a very damp area of Manitoba. The films were typical of a disease called North American blastomycosis. Our case was the first to be reported on a dog in Canada. North American blastomycosis is a fungal disease that can affect both animals and humans. The fungi are present in moist rich soil of wooded areas. Most of the cases in North America occur around the Great Lakes and Mississippi areas. The fungi are inhaled by the victim and can proliferate in various parts of the body. The disease is often found in the lungs, causing symptoms of pneumonia. Because it mimics other diseases—for example, lung cancer—it is often misdiagnosed. If a definitive diagnosis is made early enough, it can be treated with specific antibiotics.

A new client came to the office shortly after his arrival from Malta. He brought his dog, a large German shepherd, from Malta, intending to go to Vancouver on a business trip after staying a day in Toronto. The animal would accompany him. The dog exhibited a variety of unusual symptoms that included severe weight loss, anemia, cough, and eye discharge. A laboratory workup was recommended, which he said time would not permit. Although I was not comfortable with this, symptomatic treatment was started. A few days later I had a call from a Vancouver veterinarian regarding my thoughts on the case. I told him that in my opinion it was a most unusual case, probably related to exposure to some infectious disease contacted in Malta. Two weeks later the client returned with the animal. After examination I felt that the condition had greatly deteriorated. The owner was told that the dog should be referred to the Ontario Veterinary College, since I was now certain that the problem was an exotic disease and that my practice was not equipped to make the differential diagnosis.

The dog was admitted to the teaching hospital in Guelph and underwent extensive laboratory tests. An elderly veterinary parasitologist with extensive experience with tropical diseases was consulted. He called for bone marrow biopsies. When he examined the slides with a microscope, he found a tropical parasite. From this examination he was able to make the diagnosis of leishmaniasis. This disease is easily transmitted to humans and can be fatal in both animals and man. The problem was very disconcerting to the many people who had experienced contact with the dog. Fortunately there was no cross infection to any of those who had touched the animal. The dog was near death when it was referred to the Ontario Veterinary College. As soon as the diagnosis was made, and because it was considered to be highly infectious to humans, it was euthanized. The case was written up in the veterinary journals since it was the first case of the disease to be diagnosed in Canada.

Chapter Twenty-One

The Need for Qualified Help

As the new practice grew, the workload became too much for two veterinarians so we decided to employ a veterinarian, preferably one just graduating from university. In 1958 we took on a young graduate named Jim Bodendistel, a fine young man and dedicated to the profession. Jim's father was a veterinarian whom we knew. Like most young practitioners he hoped, after a year or so, to own his own business, and asked if we would consider his becoming a junior partner. I felt that he would be an ideal partner, but Dick had reservations since our own partnership was working so well and a third could complicate matters. Dick's position was understandable. He felt that we had a good partnership and that if another partner was brought in, there was a possibility of divisive "two-against-one" situations arising. I agreed. Jim decided to start on his own and asked me for advice as to a good location. I suggested the Ottawa area since there was a shortage of practitioners there. Jim took my advice and started in Ottawa. He was well liked by his clients, and because he had a lot of ability, his practice was very successful.

We had a good rapport with the Ontario Veterinary College, so when we wanted to employ a new graduate we were offered the use of the office of the head of the small animal division of the college to conduct interviews with prospective employees. A date for interviews would be set, and both of us would attend the meetings with students. We considered various factors during the interviews that would include scholastic grades, general appearance including dress, clean fingernails, ability to converse with us, and so on. We would each write our thoughts about the candidates and compare notes after the interview. These interviews occurred annually, since most new graduates used the experience in our practice as a stepping stone to starting on their own. Over the years we had a number of young graduates, most of whom, I am proud to say, have been a credit to the profession.

Chapter Twenty-Two

Speaking Engagements

Dick and I, usually working together, wrote a number of articles that were published in various veterinary publications. This often led to speaking invitations at various veterinary meetings. We both enjoyed these requests since it gave us the opportunity to repay the profession for the knowledge that had benefited us. Usually we spoke on subjects related to our own practice interests. We each had invitations to speak at local meetings in Toronto as well as at meetings of the Ontario Veterinary Association and the Canadian Veterinary Medical Association. In addition, I spoke at various local meetings in the United States as well as at annual meetings of the American Animal Hospital Association in New York, Miami, and San Francisco. I presented papers in Mexico City at a convention of the World Veterinary Association as well as papers in Australia and New Zealand.

An unusual event occurred during a seminar that I presented at the 1973 American Animal Hospital annual convention in San Francisco. The seminar was to last three hours; the subject was Geriatric Medicine. There was very little information on the subject in the veterinary journals, so most of my information came either from discussions with other practitioners or from my own observations. I had made slides to illustrate the material to be presented. Barbara was with me at he convention, and I arranged seating for her at the presentation. At midpoint, coffee was served outside the entrance to the lecture hall. I asked Barbara, not known to most of the group, to listen in on the conversation and try to get the reaction to my presentation.

Invariably attendees surround the lecturer during the coffee break to ask specific questions. Just before resuming the seminar, I had a chance to ask Barbara what she had heard. She told me that there were no derogatory remarks and lots of interest in the material. When I opened the slide projector to continue the meeting, there was a note inside which stated: "Dr. Graham, your material is substantially below my intellectual capacity." When material such as this seminar is prepared, it should be directed at the average individual as opposed to the brightest person in the audience. Somewhat disconcerted, I quickly made a decision to read the note to the group of some two hundred people. A brooding silence occurred. Reaching for my wallet, I offered to reimburse the individual his entrance fee. There was no reply to my offer, and the program was completed.

This meeting of the American Animal Hospital Association (AAHA), an organization that I described earlier, is a voluntary organization whose members consist of many veterinarians who wish to provide the best quality care for their patients. Membership is widespread throughout the world; veterinarians from other countries attended this meeting. The president announced that a special and unusual award had been made to a veterinarian named Alf Wight. He mentioned that while most of those present might not recognize him by this name, they

Sow's Ear to Silk Purse

would undoubtedly recognize him by his pen name, (James Herriot) He concluded that while the association had extended an invitation for him to attend this meeting and offered to provide all expenses for his trip, Dr. Wight replied that he could not spare the time to attend because of the pressure of his practice. After the meeting, the association sent representatives to England to make the award personally. It was fitting that this organization recognized the outstanding literary work of Alf Wight as a major public-relations contribution to our profession.

James Herriot's first two books, published in 1973 as one volume in the USA, entitled *All Creatures Great and Small,* became an overnight sensation in the USA and in England. He followed the initial books with several others, all of which enjoyed literary success. His books, as well as the television series adapted from the books, were followed worldwide not only by the public but also by the veterinary profession. His stories about animals and their owners were charming. Descriptions of the country that surrounded his practice were fascinating. He made the point that while he had little financial recompense for his efforts as a veterinarian, he enjoyed his profession. Often his accounts were not paid, and he was reluctant to chase his clients for overdue bills. This reminded me of one time when, on the fourth statement on an account, I scribbled on the bill, "Please put me in the hat with your other statements so at least I have a chance to be paid." The cheque for the account in full came by return mail.

Most veterinarians agree that James Herriot was a credit to veterinarians everywhere. We all have seen cases similar to those that he described but do not have the ability to describe them as well.

Following this convention, a colleague of mine, Dr. Bill Jackson from Lakeland Florida, and I had been invited to go to Australia and New Zealand to put on a series of educational meetings for the local veterinarians. I had known Bill for many years through professional meetings. He had spoken to our group in Toronto on several occasions and was highly regarded in the profession. Our wives were invited as well, and we received a moderate honorarium to help with the costs of the trip. Our first stop was in Sydney, followed by a tour of the area. After completing our engagements in Australia, we flew to New Zealand and spent two weeks there. Bill's wife, also named Barbara, is an enchanting lady. Born in the state of Georgia she still has that wonderful southern accent. We rented an automobile and toured most of the two islands. It was a wonderful experience.

During the internship in California, I found that some veterinarians had started practices that specialized in the feline species and limited their practices to the care and treatment of cats. This seemed unusual to a farm boy, since barn cats had little monetary value save for their usefulness in rodent control. Veterinarians rarely were paid to treat a sick or injured farm cat.

A married couple arrived with a cat that had been struck by a car. This accident resulted in a fractured femur. The repair of the injury required bone surgery. I quoted a fee of $50.00 for the surgery and the postoperative care. The man was indignant with the thought of spending this much on a worthless cat (his words). His wife promptly stated that she wanted the repair done. If he insisted on destruction of the cat, she concluded, the husband would find permanent accommodation in the spare bedroom. Because of this powerful argument, the fracture was repaired.

Perhaps the antagonism many men have towards cats has to do with their reluctance to accept domination by humans. Dogs can be trained to do tricks, act as working or guard dogs, and provide many other useful functions. Cats, on the other hand, do as they please and ignore their owners or ask to be admired as their moods dictate.

I learned a lot from the above incident and occasionally used her threat to convince reluctant male clients that their wives'

131

feline friends were important and they would gain or lose a lot of goodwill with their wives depending on their attitude.

In 1963 Dr. Jim Archibald, head of the Department of Small Animals at the Ontario Veterinary College, asked me to present a two-day seminar on feline diseases at the Maritime meeting in Moncton, New Brunswick. I had offered shorter presentations on this subject at various local meetings in Ontario. At that time there was no textbook on the subject, so most of the material was from my own experience. Jim made me an offer; if I would do the presentation he would have his staff type the notes, provided that he could use my material for class instruction at the college. I accepted his offer. I offer that part of my seminar that addresses general philosophy of the subject but does not include the actual description of and recommended treatment for the various feline disease problems. My object in presenting the seminar was to convince my audience that many clients own cats and expect their veterinarians to be competent in their care. The opening remarks of the seminar were entitled *"Client Impressions and Economics of Feline Practice"* and was presented as follows:

The first contact between the client and the veterinarian is normally by telephone. It is basic, therefore, that whoever is on telephone duty have a courteous and pleasant voice. The client feels that if the secretary is pleasant and helpful, then it would follow that the professional staff will be the same. The secretary should be able to give a limited amount of information, such as basic fees, the necessity for stool examination, and the importance of vaccination. The secretary should not make a tentative diagnosis, prescribe diets, or in general "play doctor." The doctor should talk to the client, in many instances, before seeing the patient. The efficiency of the establishment is demonstrated by the interest of the entire staff, and if the veterinarian cannot answer the telephone immediately, he or she should return the call as soon as possible.

The secretary should know that many cat owners, particularly older women, are fastidious and should encourage them to make an appointment when the office is quiet and not when there is likely to be a reception room full of dogs. In order to determine whether or not parasites are a problem, the secretary will encourage the owner to bring a sample of the animal's stool for microscopic examination and will have this set up for the doctor to examine.

Courtesy and concern shown on the telephone should again be demonstrated when the client arrives. The animal's history file will be pulled or a new file started if it is a first visit. Particular attention should be given to the spelling of the names of the pet and of the owner as well as the correct address and telephone number. If the case has been referred by another veterinarian or by another client, this should be recorded on the file card. The secretary should record on a separate piece of paper the reason for the visit. This outline should be presented to the doctor so that he or she can peruse it prior to seeing the patient. If it is a new client the secretary should formally introduce the client to the doctor. The doctor should have a neat, professional appearance: hair groomed and the nails clean. The client will rightly or wrongly form an impression of the establishment and of the veterinarian within the first minute that will include an opinion of the personality of the doctor as well as ability with and knowledge of cats. The client may have been referred because of the reputation as an expert in feline medicine.

The ability of the veterinarian is demonstrated by the method of restraint, the voice used, and the ability to reassure the cat and the client. Cats should not be handled roughly during restraint; furthermore, the client is likely to be upset if this type of restraint is used. If the cat is upset, it should be restrained by sedation or by anaesthesia.

Before and during the examination, information should be recorded on the file card, as an accurate history is essential in feline medicine. If at this stage of the examination the diagnosis is obvious, the client should be so informed and the method or methods of handling the problem discussed with the client. Veterinarians occasionally tend to be evasive and undermine the intelligence of the owner. If the diagnosis is not obvious, this should be stated. The client should then be told what steps, such as hematology, radiology, or urinalysis, will be needed to clarify the problem. An estimate should be given at this time as to the costs involved for this investigational work, and it should be explained that after the final diagnosis has been made the prognosis and final cost will be estimated. There will, of course, be clients who will prefer that the patient be treated symptomatically rather than undergo the expense of a proper investigation. It is surprising that when the problem is properly presented many clients will want good work done rather than have inadequate management of the case.

A minimum of fifteen minutes should be allocated for the examination and discussion. At the conclusion of the discussion, the cat should be picked up properly and the client dismissed by opening the door of the examination room and told that the results of the investigational work will be communicated by telephone at a specific time. This telephone call should be followed by a daily progress report for the duration of the animal's stay. This report should be made by the veterinarian—not by the secretary or by the animal attendant. When the animal is released, the veterinarian should give specific instructions to be carried out during convalescence; i.e., expected duration of recovery, the type of medication to *be used with instructions how it should be administered, special diets if necessary, and the date on which sutures should be removed if applicable. The account should be itemized and presented by the veterinarian so that if there are any questions about the account they can be answered by the veterinarian rather than by the secretary. If the client has been properly prepared during the hospital stay, there will seldom be a query of the amount. An appointment should be made for any further treatments. The client should be told that a telephone call would be appreciated if any problems arise. Mention should be made of any prophylactic therapy, such as vaccines, which would be deemed advisable in the future.*

Do not forget that cat owners will be more observant, more critical, and more loyal than other clients provided that interest and ability to deal with their problems is apparent.

The Necessity for Sterile Surgery

As recently as fifteen years ago, only exceptional veterinarians performed sterile surgery. As a profession we are fortunate that the poor work carried out in the operating theatre by some of our members has not degraded the whole profession. The day is fast approaching when it will be an offence punishable by suspension of licence to practice to operate contrary to accepted principles. The procedures and techniques used in our surgeries should be of a quality that we would insist on in treatments by our medical friends. It would be unthinkable for a surgeon to explore the abdomen of a human with bare hands after performing a rectal examination or opening an abscess, yet animal patients are often exposed to such an indignity. The following are some of the reasons why inadequate surgical technique is carried out in some veterinary establishments:

1. Inadequate fees to warrant doing a good procedure.

2. Absence of progressive ideas. "I've gotten along without too much trouble over the years; why change?"

3. Disinclination because of cost to provide adequate equipment such as autoclave, oxygen apparatus, even drapes and gloves.

4. Losing an animal undergoing surgery means very little to a veterinarian with no conscience or professional pride.

5. Some veterinarians state that they cannot palpate tissues effectively through rubber gloves.

6. It has been stated that there are a few veterinarians who would suffer a curtailed income since iatrogenic illnesses such as osteomyelitis would seldom be seen.

7. Some veterinarians do not realize that they are open to legal action if inferior surgery should result in incapacity, deformity, or death. They have not done what a prudent veterinary surgeon would have done under the same circumstances.

Handling and Restraint of Cats

Cats are presented for examination in all manner of containers, from potato sacks and cardboard boxes to more adequate containers, such as plywood carrying cases especially built for the purpose. Frequently the owner will request advice as to what would be a suitable container. It should be suggested that a box hinged so that the top turns back would be preferable to a case with a small hole at the end through which the cat has to be extracted. Several half-inch holes should be drilled at the end of the case to provide ventilation. A wicker picnic basket makes an adequate and convenient carrying case. Relative darkness in the carrying case is preferable to a well-lit case, since limited light makes the cat feel more secure.

Speaking Engagements

When the cat is to be removed from the case, a noise should be made near the bottom of the case that will attract its attention. The case is then opened and the cat is grasped firmly by the scruff of the neck with the left hand and with the right hand by the base of the tail and by the hind legs near the stifle joints. The cat is then placed quickly on the examination table and released. If at this time the shoulders and back are stroked gently and firmly, the animal will usually stay where it was placed. Firm pressure over the shoulders and loins will quietly subdue the animal if it is still restless. The owner can be instructed to follow these procedures while the veterinarian is making the examination or administering an injection. In most cases a small amount of pressure will make the cat feel that it cannot escape and therefore it will remain quiet and comfortable.

Recent graduates are likely to purchase a canvas cat bag. Only a limited amount of experience is necessary to reveal the futility of this purchase. If the cat is so wild that it cannot be restrained by the above methods, it should be sedated or given a general anaesthetic. Rolling a cat in a blanket for castration is barbarous. Many clients will ask if the animal will be anaesthetized during a surgical procedure and must be reassured as to the humane treatment it will receive.

Cat owners often complain that their previous veterinarian dispensed tablets for treatment of some problem but gave no instruction as to the method of administration of the medication or that the tablets were too large to administer easily. One useful method is as follows: Have an assistant place the index fingers around the elbow joints and the thumbs on the shoulders, at the same time exerting downward pressure with the thumbs. The person administering the tablet takes the head of the cat firmly in the left hand and tips the head upward.

The tablet is then placed between the thumb and index finger of the right hand. The second finger of the right hand is placed between the lower canine teeth. The mouth usually opens readily as slight upward pressure with the left hand and slight downward pressure with the right index finger is applied. The tablet is dropped over the root of the tongue and the mouth is closed. If the tablet is not placed deeply over the root of the tongue, it can be pushed downward with a stab of the right index finger or with the eraser of a lead pencil. Swallowing is facilitated if the tablet has been coated with butter or mineral oil and if the throat is stroked as soon as the mouth has been closed. There is little excuse for anyone to be scratched if the procedure is carried out in the proper manner. A moment spent demonstrating this procedure to the owner is always appreciated.

The owner also appreciates a demonstration of the proper method to carry a cat. The right middle finger is placed between the elbows of the cat with the thumb and the remainder of the hand on the outside of the elbows. The pelvis of the cat is then placed under the right arm and firm pressure is exerted, which pushes the cat against the ribs of the person restraining it. The cat is quite comfortable and doesn't struggle. If the cat is to be carried past a dog, the person carrying the cat should keep the body between the cat's eyes and the dog.

If owners are scratched or bitten by their own animals on the premises of a veterinarian because of fright, the practitioner may be legally liable.

Occasionally a cat is so nervous that it may be difficult to remove from its kennel. In such cases a large towel or blanket dropped over the animal will placate it, probably because it cannot see the person of whom it is afraid. The cat may then be picked up through the towel. Such cats should be given an injectable tranquilizer.

Only an experienced attendant should handle a cat of this nature. Inexperience of the handler will augment the anxiety of such an animal.

Handouts of the material of about eighty typewritten pages, including this preamble as well as description of and treatment for various feline diseases, were given to each attending veterinarian. Almost all of the attendees felt that they could improve their management of cat problems after the meeting.

Chapter Twenty-Three

Emergencies

Contemporary veterinary practitioners in urban areas rarely provide after-hours emergency service for their clients. Most cities now have specialized veterinary emergency clinics to provide it, and most individual practices refer their cases to these clinics that were started about the same time that I left active practice. At the Amherst Clinic, if an after-hours emergency arose, whichever of our own veterinarians was on call had his own backup staff to assist with procedure. The following two cases presented exceptions.

Emergency procedures, often after normal office hours, were frequent and often difficult to manage, especially if our own backup people were not available. The following illustrates such a problem. When Janet was about eight years old, we received a call asking for assistance for a dog in labour. The owner was not a regular client and his own veterinarian was unavailable. Nor were my own people available to help. When I examined the animal, a large boxer, I determined that she could not have a normal delivery and required caesarean section. I phoned Barbara and asked her to assist me and to bring Janet.

I induced the animal with an intravenous anaesthetic and prepared the surgical area. An endotracheal tube was inserted, and we were ready for surgery. Using ether, Barbara maintained the anaesthetic while I performed the operation. Removing the puppies one by one from the uterus, I tossed them to Janet, who caught them in a towel. For stimulation she massaged them until breathing was established. There were nine puppies in the litter, all of which survived.

A Great Dane, again owned by the client of another veterinarian, turned up for emergency treatment on a holiday weekend, and again our own staff was unavailable for backup assistance. The problem in this animal was torsion of the stomach, invariably fatal if not quickly corrected surgically. I was desperate for the hands of another surgeon to assist with this difficult procedure. I phoned my good friend and former employee Dr. Ken Gadd, now working in another practice. He agreed to assist. Torsion of the stomach is occasionally seen in large, deep-chested dogs soon after they have eaten a large meal and indulged in excessive exercise. The stomach flips over, and gas formation trapped there results in extreme bloating. Ken and I were able to turn the stomach back to its normal position and empty its contents. I was very thankful for Ken's assistance. Without it, the dog would have been lost.

About a week later the owner brought the animal back for removal of sutures. He did not appear thankful that the dog was still alive. After I had removed the sutures, he said that I had conned him for what at that time was a large fee and that there was no such disease as torsion of the stomach. When I inquired where he had obtained this advice, he told me that his regular veterinarian had informed him that there was no such problem. Annoyed that he had been given this misinformation, I asked him to come to my office and to listen to a telephone conversation. I put through a call to Dr. Jim Archibald at the Ontario Veterinary College and outlined the case. Jim asked to speak to the client and told him that in fact such a problem existed, that he was fortunate that his regular veterinarian was unavailable, and that our efforts had saved the life of the dog. The client was most apologetic. I phoned the other veterinarian and suggested that he upgrade his knowledge.

I wonder if this man was the kind of person that his dog thought he was. If the dog thought he was above reproach, he may have been mistaken and given undue credit to his owner!

Sometimes what seems to be an emergency may be something very simple. About two a.m. one morning I was awakened by a call for assistance from a man known to me as a high-powered businessman. I had been told by a mutual acquaintance that he liked to try to intimidate anyone with whom he dealt. The dog in question arrived with the owner as well as his wife. A large amount of saliva was escaping from the mouth of the animal, the lower jaw hanging down. The animal was bright and alert. Since dumb rabies was a distinct possibility, I put on a pair of rubber gloves before attempting to examine the mouth and throat. With the mouth widely opened, the diagnosis was obvious; a pork chop bone was caught on both sides of the upper molars! It was easily removed with forceps. The owner, who appeared to have consumed a substantial amount of liquid libation, asked me the fee. I told him that the office visit was ten dollars with an additional ten dollars for the after-hours service. He became quite belligerent.

I replied, "You have to make one of two choices: either forget the fee altogether and never come back to this office or pay the fee and apologize for your outburst." He chose the latter option. That was his last complaint about my service.

Again, it would be interesting to speculate on the dog's opinion of his master, since this man was not highly thought of by his friends.

Chapter Twenty-Four

Bad Dogs

Like owners who are not polite and trustworthy, dogs on occasion exhibit aggressive behaviour. The following illustrate the point.

A six-week-old cocker spaniel was brought to my office for routine vaccinations. The aggressive puppy attempted to bite. I informed the owner that this unusual behaviour should not be tolerated. He laughed at my concerns. Each time the animal was presented, it became more aggressive and further advice was given to the owner concerning the misbehaviour. The owner continued to ignore my concerns. When the dog attained the age of eighteen months, the owner began to have concerns since it had bitten the child of a neighbour. Since this was the last client of the evening, I suggested that we sit in my reception area to further discuss the matter. The owner sat beside me with the dog between us. The owner's hand was hanging down close to the head of the dog. Suddenly, without provocation, the dog attacked the hand, inflicting deep wounds on both sides. The owner looked at the damage and said, "I wish that I had listened to you in the beginning." He then asked that the animal be destroyed.

A next-door neighbour at our cottage, a lawyer, had an elderly Great Dane that I had seen on a few occasions. This animal had behaved well all of its life. It eventually died in its sleep at the residence of the owner. Soon after he acquired another Great Dane, this time a puppy. Similar to the cocker spaniel, the Dane was very aggressive as a juvenile. Again my friend the lawyer laughed at my concerns. The same pattern emerged as the dog grew older. Each time the dog was presented, its disposition seemed to get worse. Finally one evening when the dog was about two years old, he brought the dog in for a routine matter. The owner stayed in the reception area while I examined the dog. This time the dog tried to jump at my throat. Fortunately I was able to slide the examination table between us. Carefully, I slid a rope over the neck of the animal to restrain it. I led it into the reception area to discuss the case with the owner.

"Albert, this dog doesn't like me, and I don't like him. Because he is so large and so potentially dangerous, he should be destroyed before he kills someone. If you do not accept this advice, you will have to find another veterinarian to look after him. Furthermore, should you keep him and he does attack someone—and this is highly probable—I could be called as an expert witness. I would then be obliged to divulge the advice which has been given to you." No doubt because of his legal training, Albert immediately accepted my advice.

One morning I read in the local newspaper that a Doberman that I had seen once or twice had attacked and killed the child of the family. According to the newspaper, the owner of the dog, a woman, picked up her husband's shotgun and killed the animal in her living room with one blast. A few months later she arrived in my office with another puppy and announced to my waiting room full of people that she was the

lady who had shot the dog that had killed her child. It is difficult to comprehend the lack of sensitivity displayed by this person. I have often wondered whether if she had recognized that
she had a problem animal, the death of the child could have
been prevented. If she had known that the dog was not trustworthy, she should have provided better supervision when it
was with the child. While I did not enjoy destroying a healthy
dog, I have no hesitation in destroying an animal that would
attack a human, particularly a defenseless child.

There is no doubt in my mind that the three dogs described
above had forfeited their right to live in a family environment.

In certain cases euthanasia is the correct advice to be given
to the client. Owners of an animal that is terminal and suffering
because of a generalized malignancy should be given this advice.
Some owners would disagree, because the animal had been a
family member for so long. When this was the case, I would tell
them that the patient would continue to get worse and no doubt
continue to suffer. I would also tell them that if they kept the
animal beyond the point where it could enjoy life, they were
being selfish to put their interest before that of their pet.

I have often thought about the laws of our country that dis-
allow the wishes of a terminal human patient who would like
to have a peaceful end to his or her life as opposed to being
required to end it on a bed of suffering, many months later,
because the medical profession has the ability to sustain life
with heroic treatment. In my case I have a legal document
called a *Living Will* that directs my executor and the attending
physicians not to keep me alive by artificial means if my case
is hopeless, especially if suffering is involved. What would be
the benefit to the patient during those last weeks or months?
Some might consider such a document to be synonymous with
suicide. I regard it as a rational action made while my brain
was capable of making such a decision.

It is not unusual for an owner to bring a perfectly healthy
animal to the office of a veterinarian and request euthanasia.

There are many reasons for such requests, some of which are described in these memoirs. I also described how most of our own animals were brought in to be euthanized for various reasons and given to me when I told the owners that I would give them a home rather than destroy them.

In other cases the owner may not be able to afford its maintenance or has simply grown tired of owning the pet that had been adopted with little consideration of its future.

When euthanasia was requested by an owner, I required his signature with respect to their decision. On one occasion a man in his forties brought a healthy dog to be destroyed. I asked why he had come to this decision; he would not give me a reason, and I could not dissuade him from it. He was distraught, tears flowing down his face. He requested that he be present when the lethal intravenous injection was made.

About two months later, three boys in their early teens arrived at the hospital to visit their pet. Their father had told them that the animal had been hospitalized for extensive treatment. After review of the in-patient files, I could find no animal under the name given. A few moments later, since the surname was unusual, I recognized it and went to the euthanasia records.

I had no reasonable choice in this unfortunate situation. I showed the document to the boys and asked them if they recognized their father's signature. The boys were devastated that their pet was dead and that their father had lied to them.

I have often thought about this incident of more than forty years ago. Had I declined to destroy the dog, would the owner have done it himself using a means that would have been more traumatic? What was the eventual psychiatric effect on the boys?

Chapter Twenty-Five

More on the Problem
of Rabies

When the problem of rabies became endemic in wildlife, particularly in skunks, raccoons, and foxes, the veterinary profession had to be alert to the possibility of its spreading to communities. Rabid animals were numerous in the Greater Toronto area and could readily infect dogs and cats.

A girl of about twelve, whose father was a good friend of mine and a client of the practice, brought in a small skunk for treatment. The skunk was very ill and seemed quite lethargic. Its lower jaw was slack and non-responsive. The girl had numerous warts on her hands, some of them open. With the possibility of rabies on my mind, I suggested that the skunk be left in hospital for observation. It died in a few hours, and I removed the head for laboratory examination. I informed the father of the circumstances and told him to notify their family physician of the problem. When the test for rabies confirmed positive, the child was started on a preventative program known as Pasteur treatment. The girl had no after-effects from the treatments that at the time consisted of one injection per day for a period of fourteen days.

A few months later several groups of men were sitting on the veranda of our golf club following the morning's golf. Suddenly the father of the girl stood up and asked for the attention of the group while he said a few words. He gave a dissertation on how, in all probability, I had saved the life of his daughter. I was overwhelmed by his words and felt that I had done no more than would most other veterinarians.

Some time after this incident, a litter of foxes was born in a culvert under the third tee of the golf club. There were four babies in the litter, and as they grew the parents seemed hard pressed to find enough food for them. I saw the female fox carrying a dead cat back to her den, returning from a southern direction where a diagnosis of a positive case of rabies in another cat had been made a few weeks previously.

I wrote the following information letter that was included in the club's monthly mailing:

To the Members—Scarboro Golf and Country Club
The directors of the club have asked me, because of my training in veterinary medicine, to prepare an information letter with respect to the resident fox population. I am sure that all of us agree that these handsome animals enhance the natural beauty of the golf course. Unfortunately, foxes as well as skunks and raccoons are the principle vectors of rabies in Ontario.

On a square mile basis, the incidence of rabies is higher in Southern Ontario than is the case anywhere in the world. For the first six months of 1986, the number of cases of humans requiring preventative treatment for the disease has increased 150 percent over the same period in 1985. It is estimated that some 4000 people in Ontario will be given preventative treatment in 1986. Several cases of rabies in animals have been confirmed recently in Scarborough. One of these confirmed cases was a stray cat that had bitten a child. This case occurred less than a mile from club property.

Rabies is caused by a virus present in the saliva of affected animals and is usually transmitted by a bite wound. Theoretically it can also be transmitted to the recipient through an open wound. The virus can be present in the saliva up to ten days prior to the onset of symptoms. The disease has two classic forms, one of which is dumb rabies and the other furious rabies. In dumb rabies the lower jaw of the victim is paralyzed and the animal salivates profusely; in furious rabies, the animal is aggressive, roams widely, and will attack other animals or humans. In their demented state, rabid foxes have been observed attacking inanimate objects such as railway tracks with ferocity sufficient to break their teeth. Rabies is one of the few diseases of animals or man where death of the victim is inevitable, usually in a few hours to two or three days after the onset of symptoms.

The foxes on club property have been observed mouthing golf balls. Since rabies virus can occur in saliva prior to the onset of symptoms, it is inadvisable for a human to handle such a ball.

On an experimental basis in remote parts of Ontario, oral rabies vaccine is being administered to foxes. The Ministry of Natural Resources hopes that if large numbers of foxes can be immunized, the incidence of the disease can be reduced. I have attempted to obtain some of this experimental vaccine for administration to foxes on the club property. Since the vaccine is still in the experimental stage for use in remote areas, I was unable to obtain a supply.

I have consulted with the Ministry of Natural Resources, the Scarborough Department of Health and the Scarborough Animal Control about our problem. All were in agreement that the foxes should be removed from the club property.

Accordingly, the board of directors of the club has engaged a firm to live-trap the animals and remove them from the club property. Since foxes are extremely intelligent, they may be difficult to trap. If they are not caught, and provided that they do not die of rabies, the probability is high that they will migrate when the existing food supply is exhausted.

Under normal circumstances, foxes are shy animals and avoid humans. One of the classic symptoms of early rabies in wild animals is loss of fear of humans. Our foxes have lost their natural timidity because of close association with humans. In my opinion this poses a serious problem. Should one of these foxes develop furious rabies, it would attack an unsuspecting golfer from close range.

As long as foxes are on club property, it should be incumbent upon every golfer to have a club in hand with which to defend himself should one of these foxes show signs of aggression.

Yours truly,

J.E.B. Graham DVM

Response by members of the club to this information letter was considerable. A club member, whose husband was a member as well as being a practising physician in the area, telephoned me. She said that, while she always advised her children to avoid wild animals, she was one of those who played with golf balls that the little foxes had mouthed. Her words were: "How could I have been so stupid?" Two other members told me that they had played at other golf courses, one in British Columbia and one in Florida. Both courses had copies of my letter posted in their locker rooms. It seems that the advice was timely and well accepted. The foxes were successfully live-trapped and taken elsewhere.

Chapter Twenty-Six

Home Life

When Janet was a year old, Barbara and I decided that we should increase the size of our family. Two years of trying produced no pregnancy. We sought professional help and had many tests to find the reason. No explanation was forthcoming. I often wondered if either my exposure to X-ray radiation or her fibroids was the problem, but neither was ever substantiated. Eventually we accepted that Janet would be an only child and felt fortunate that we at least had one wonderful offspring.

Janet's public school was a short walk from our home, so she was able to return for lunch. Our new hospital was also quite close to our home, so lunch with my family was possible on most days. Since evening office hours often precluded dinners together, our lunches together were important.

Janet loved her animals. Our dog Pete was her buddy, and she delighted in his company. Often she would make believe that he was a horse and put a set of straps on his shoulders so that she could pretend to drive him. As time progressed she decided that she would like to have another pet, preferably a cat. Our first cat was a white part Persian that she named Frosty. Frosty's previous owner brought him in for destruction since the owner had grown tired of him. I did not like to kill a healthy animal and offered to adopt him, to which the owner immediately agreed. He was a male cat who had an intense dislike of dogs. In the beginning Frosty and Pete avoided each other, but as time progressed they became friends.

The next adoption, under the same circumstances, was a five-month Siamese cat who was given the name "Henry." Henry met a sad fate in that he disappeared. Later we were told that a neighbour had killed him. His replacement was another Siamese, this time given to me because the owner's child was allergic to the cat. I brought her home during lunch hour. Janet welcomed her and picked her up. Unfortunately the kitten, that we named Sheba, became frightened and scratched Janet's lip with her sharp kitten claws. Blood flowed extensively. Janet insisted that it was not the fault of the kitten and begged that we keep her. Of course we agreed.

Sheba was a house cat and except for two occasions never left the house. One evening when she was about two years old, she escaped through an open door. A neighbour came to the door and said that he had found an injured cat on the street. I said to phone the hospital since it was not my night on call. I then looked at the animal and discovered that it was Sheba. A car had struck her. Examination at the hospital revealed that she had a badly fractured jaw. I repaired the jaw with surgical wire. Since the cat was a sensitive animal, we decided that she would be better at home. We had to force-feed her, to which she objected. Two days later she started to vomit, so I took her back for further examination. I found that one of her kidneys had been ruptured by the automobile trauma. My surgical intervention revealed that the kidney could not be repaired. I had no option but to remove it. She lived for twelve more years with one kidney. The second time she escaped from our home she was attacked, and killed, by a dog.

Home Life

When Janet was in the final year of public school, rumours circulated regarding the use of illicit drugs in the high schools. Concerned, Barbara and I discussed means of averting the problem as far as our daughter was concerned. The solution we arrived at produced advantages extending beyond her high school years. My old friend Roly Armitage was involved in the racehorse industry. One of his clients owned a three-year-old standard-bred mare. She had been trained and raced prior to the time that her leg bones were properly developed. She became lame and unable to perform at an acceptable level. We purchased the mare with the understanding that with moderate exercise she would not be lame and could be a riding horse. The name of the horse was Miss Jan Direct. She was a quiet, well-mannered animal. We found a horse-boarding farm in Pickering, a few miles east of our home, and the horse was taken to this establishment. Janet, as most young girls would be, was very happy to be associated with a horse. The rules were strict in that she was expected to be responsible for the care of the horse, including cleaning the barn and grooming the animal. Either Barbara or I would drive her to the stable on weekends to attend to her responsibilities. She received riding lessons and became a competent rider.

She enjoyed the experience and eventually competed in a variety of equestrian events acquiring numerous ribbons. Her activities, as we expected, kept her much too busy to associate with individuals who could have led her astray. From time to time the horse was transferred to other establishments. Our friends the Harris family rented a farmhouse on 100 acres a few miles north of our home. They offered the use of the barn for Jan's horse, and we accepted the offer. When Jan was old enough to get her driver's licence, she was able to make the trips to see her horse without our assistance. She owned the horse until it was more than twenty years old. Eventually arthritis in the horse's legs that resulted from the early training necessitated euthanasia.

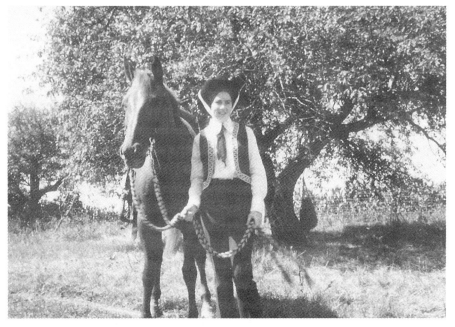

Jan and Horse

The students of Wellesley School of Nursing, graduation year 1949, were close friends during their training. Following graduation their friendship persevered. Once monthly, rain or shine, these ladies would get together, usually at the home of one of them. Sometimes the husbands were invited as well to one of the homes, usually in smaller groups, for a dinner party. The association of these ladies, those who are still alive, continues. If one of these ladies had a problem the rest were willing to help in any way possible. Barbara's classmates were staunch supporters throughout her long illness.

From time to time after she was in high school, we called on Janet to provide temporary secretarial assistance at our hospital. One Saturday I was on duty with another veterinarian when a client came in for a consultation. Janet asked which doctor the client wished to see. Not knowing that she was my daughter, the client said, "Anybody but Dr. Graham." You can't win them all! I found out after looking at our records that this client was delinquent in paying a long overdue account. I guess that he had did not want me to confront him with the outstanding bill.

Janet's maternal grandparents, Walter and Eldora Baldwin, were retired, and when Janet was an infant were happy to babysit and let us get away for a brief holiday. As she got older they would visit frequently, often staying for a meal. Walter enjoyed a glass of rye, about which his wife was not enthusiastic. He developed a routine that allowed him to enjoy his drink without being caught. As soon as they arrived, he would make a cup of tea. While Barbara and her mother were talking, Walter would sneak down to the bar, dump the tea, and replace it with rye. Since the liquids were essentially the same colour, he got away with it for years.

Eldora and Walter were snowbirds and spent most of their winters in the southern United States. Frequently they invited us to visit their winter home for a week or more. When the pressures of practice precluded my presence, Barbara would take Janet and spend a week with her parents. One year the three of us visited the grandparents in their rental home at Daytona Beach, Florida. The access to the beach was down a flight of stairs from the cottage. Walter had volunteered to babysit (Janet was three years old) while we went for a walk. He dozed off, and Janet wandered out on the beach. She knew that the access steps to the cottage were painted green, but when she tried to find her way back all of the steps to the row of cottages were also painted green. After a frantic search, we found her wandering along the wide beach in search of the correct green steps.

My in-laws were wonderful people. We enjoyed many visits at their home, our home, and on a few occasions drove together to my parents' home on the family farm. Barbara's mother, before she was married, had been a milliner. She taught Barbara her art as well as the art of dressmaking. This became a hobby for Barbara, and eventually she designed and made most of her own attire. She received many compliments for her original clothing designs.

During my early practice years in Ontario, I had faithfully paid my annual fees to the state of California to maintain my licence. Eventually I wondered if this was a mistake since there was no indication that we would ever return. A few years later I decided that the licence should be regained since it was automatically revoked when the payments stopped. I inquired to determine what steps were necessary to have the license reinstated. The requirements were as follows: clearance from the local police department, including the taking of finger-prints, to ensure that there had been no criminal convictions, letters of reference from various people and institutions includ-ing my Alma Mater, a list of contributions made to the profes-sion, speeches that been made to colleagues as well as papers published in the professional journals. I had sent programs related to the various speeches that I had made to my mother and father and these records were still available. When all of this material was sent to California, my license was reinstated. I never used it.

In April 1965, the Baldwins were returning from a winter in Florida. On northbound Interstate Highway 75 they had a terrible accident that resulted in the death of Walter Baldwin. Eldora phoned me from the hospital in Adele, Georgia, near the scene of the accident. She knew that her husband was dead and that she had severe injuries. I told her that we would be there as soon as possible. Barbara was distraught with the news. The parents of one of Janet's school friends offered to look after Janet during our absence. We flew to New York and caught a connecting flight to Atlanta, arriving at midnight. After an overnight stay in Atlanta we took another flight to Valdosta, Georgia, where we rented a car for the trip to Adele.

Eldora had numerous lacerations on her face as well as on various parts of her body. These had been surgically repaired. She had the presence of mind to tell the hospital staff of instructions that Walter had given her many years before. He had been a Mason and had risen through the chairs to their highest level. He had told Eldora if she were in desperate need of help to notify the Masonic organization. She had always kept the ring that identified his status in the organization on her person. We arrived about twenty-four hours after the accident. By this time the Masonic organization had been most helpful. The head surgeon of the hospital who had attended her was a Mason, as were the undertaker, the local veterinarian, the local car dealer who offered us free use of a car (which we declined since we had a rental), and the local sheriff. Each of these people offered great help. The sheriff, for example, personally took us to the scene of the accident to explain how it had happened. He even provided me with a copy of the official investigative findings.

The head surgeon invited us to his home where he and his wife put on a splendid dinner for us. As we were finishing, the phone rang and he was required to return to the hospital. He asked me to come. It seems that two men had been fighting with straight razors and that one had a severe neck injury. It turned out that both the jugular vein and the carotid artery on the neck of one of the men was exposed but not damaged. The man was very fortunate to survive.

The automobile was only a few months old at the time of the accident. The impact of hitting an oak tree at eighty miles an hour, as stated in the accident report, bent the frame on both sides so badly that it resembled a "Z." The insurance adjuster examining the vehicle wanted to have it repaired, whereas I felt that it should be written off. When he wouldn't accept my position, I asked the sheriff for his opinion. "Leave it with me," he said. The next day the adjuster phoned to say that he had changed his mind and that he now believed that the car should not be repaired.

About a week after the accident, Eldora was ready to be taken home. Since she was still most uncomfortable, we arranged for a private plane to pick us up in Adele and take us to Toronto. Prior to takeoff about twelve people from the hospital came to the airport to wish us well on the return flight. Walter's body had been prepared by the local undertaker and had been sent to an undertaking parlour close to the Baldwin residence.

Over the years I have heard a lot of derogatory comments regarding the Masonic Order. This incident demonstrates the care and consideration shown during our period of grief.

Sunday evenings we usually had dinner together, and as Janet got older we would discuss many things, including what she would like to do at university. As she approached the end of high school, she frequently expressed an interest in becoming a veterinarian. I tried to dissuade her from the profession since it necessitates long hours and imposes lots of stress. It was my opinion that the profession tended to coarsen a female. I told her about a female classmate of mine who decided to start a large-animal practice and wondered why she quickly developed a busy practice related to cattle obstetrics. One old farmer told her that it was much more exciting for them to see a lady veterinarian strip to her brassiere and deliver a calf than it was to see a male strip to the waist.

Eventually Janet made the decision to enter Queen's University at Kingston, Ontario, and take the degree course which would lead to the "Bachelor of Science Nursing" degree. This course required four years to complete, with her graduation to occur in May, 1975. We felt that this study would be more suitable for her than would veterinary medicine. It left us with the hope that she might continue studies and enter medicine.

We rented a trailer to transport her furniture to Kingston and found a suitable apartment that she shared with some of her female classmates. I must say that both her mother and I felt lonely now that our offspring had left the nest.

Her four years at university were a great learning experience insofar as understanding some of the problems related to the human body is concerned. I have no doubt that this experience was very helpful during her undergraduate years in medicine. Nurses are trained to look after the basic needs of patients. The prevention of bedsores (decubitus ulcers) is an example as is the ability to monitor various body functions, perhaps to a greater degree than would a physician in training.

On days off she would frequently bring one or more of her classmates for a visit to our home and often she would visit the parents of her classmates as well. Janet still is in contact with some of these friends from years gone by. In addition Barbara and I, when time permitted, would make the two-hour trip to visit her in Kingston.

Janet had a high school boyfriend named Glen Scott. They continued to see each other when she came home for a visit. This lad studied engineering at the University of Toronto and graduated from university the same year that Janet completed her training at Queen's.

A large party attended Janet's graduation: her grandparents, her mother's sister Evelyn and her husband Steve, and, of course, Barbara and I. It was a proud day for all in attendance to see these pretty young ladies receive their recognition for four years of hard work.

After graduation Janet obtained a position as an emergency room nurse at North York General Hospital. This was a shift-work job, a very stressful position. She lived at home with us and travelled back and forth to work in the new car we had given as a graduation present. Despite the life-and-death atmosphere of a busy emergency hospital unit, she enjoyed the work that gave her the opportunity of putting to use some of the things she had studied. When we had the opportunity, we often discussed comparative medicine.

Chapter Twenty-Seven

The Decision to
Leave Active Practice

Between 1958 and 1969, the Amherst Veterinary Hospital had a succession of young veterinarians who wanted to upgrade their skills by working in our practice. After a year or so most of them started their own businesses. With few exceptions, all of them were a credit to our profession. In 1969 we brought two new graduates into our practice, Dr. McLeod and Dr. Stonehouse. As usual, we interviewed them at the college, and we agreed that they both would become assets to the practice. In time we continued to feel that both had the capability of becoming permanent fixtures in our organization. As usual, they approached us to become partners. We felt that the time had come to have more stability in the professional staff and decided to draw up a partnership agreement. This was accomplished by a good legal firm that produced a document some twenty pages in length. The financial terms and the purchase price were substantially more beneficial to the junior partners than to

Dick and to me. To facilitate the purchase, the buyout and payout to us was to take place over several years.

Dr. Holt Webster, a long time friend, was ready to retire in 1973 and offered to sell his Oshawa practice to our group. After proper evaluation by an independent appraiser, the terms and conditions of the purchase were set. The transaction completed, one of the juniors, Dr. McLeod, took over the operation. This left Dr. Ketchell, Dr. Stonehouse, and me to operate the Amherst Veterinary Hospital. The four partners would have a monthly management meeting to discuss the operation of the two practices. Invariably the idea of a substantial increase in fee structure would recur. In the beginning Dick was on my side of the argument, but he came to accept the ideas of the juniors. I was still adamant that the fees should be kept at a moderate level, as had always been the case. Now the situation was exactly as Dick had predicted many years before when we rejected the idea of Dr. Bodendistel becoming a partner. I was disappointed that the Amherst Veterinary Hospital, built on the foundation of fees affordable to most clients, was about to change its philosophy.

The situation became untenable, and after due consideration I had to face reality. Either I would buy out the other partners or offer my partnership share to them pursuant to the provisions of our agreement. I chose the latter and offered my share to the others, who accepted the terms. My years in active veterinary medicine ended in the middle of May 1975.

Barbara was devastated by the turn of events. She believed, as did I, that the terms given to the purchase of an interest by the younger partners had been much too lenient. In addition, since I had always prided myself on being a good judge of character, I knew in retrospect I had made a bad mistake.

There is an old saying: "Enjoy the setbacks, too; you can learn more from mistakes than you ever can from successes.

The business equivalent of a two-by-four right between the eyes can be one of the best learning experiences." It would be fair to say that my second career was more profitable than were my years as a practising veterinarian.

SECTION FOUR

A New Career

Chapter Twenty-Eight

A New Career

Both Barbara and I had an interest in real-estate investments and had made several purchases and sales, all of which had produced capital gains. During the winter of 1974-1975, we decided to upgrade our knowledge of real estate by taking a course at one of the community colleges in our area. This course was designed to extend information about the subject of selling and to train participants to become salespeople. We enjoyed the course, and both of us passed the examinations. Little did I know that a few months later I would make use of those real estate lectures to leave active practice and start a new career.

When the subject of a possible investment arose, whether in real estate or in the stock market, we would always discuss it with each other. If one of us dissented, the matter was always closed. The moderate fee structure coupled with the high volume practice allowed some funds to accrue as savings. Neither of us wanted a luxurious living, so the savings grew and were invested. We were firm believers in the "Rule of

Seventy-two" that states that when an interest factor is divided into seventy-two, it gives the number of years necessary for the investment to double. For example, if a 10 percent interest factor is divided into seventy-two, the investment doubles in 7.2 years. Obviously, if the original capital is spent, there is no capital to double. This is a problem with many young people today; rather than save for the future they spend their money, leaving no capital to grow.

When I left the practice in May, we made the decision to spend the summer at our cottage on Kennesis Lake in Haliburton County. This gave us a lot of time to think and to plan for the future. Toward the end of the summer, I made the decision to utilize the real-estate training recently acquired. The idea occurred to me that there was nobody in Canada qualified to evaluate the business of veterinary practices and to act as the selling agent for veterinarians. Although I knew a good deal about the real-estate part of veterinary medicine, I needed more experience. I applied and was accepted as a salesman in the commercial division of a company known at that time as A. E. Lepage (now known as Royal Lepage), located in mid Toronto. This company was involved in the sales and leasing of many types of commercial properties. I gained good experience from this employment, especially in the field of financing. My sales associates, as well as the manager of the office, were most helpful in upgrading my knowledge.

On December 22, 1975, about two months after I had joined Lepage, I retired earlier than usual since some chest discomfort had occurred. About 1:00 a.m. on the 23rd, I awoke with severe chest pain, which radiated down one arm. There was no question that something serious was happening, but I felt that it would pass. Instead, the discomfort quickly worsened. Barbara was concerned and asked Janet to see me. Janet had just finished the evening shift in the emergency room of her hospital. She suspected, as did I, that a coronary thrombosis had occurred, and she called an ambulance. She wanted to take me to her hospital, but since my condition was rapidly deteriorating she elected to stop at another, closer, hospital. The staff at Scarborough General Hospital immediately put me in critical care and attached me to a variety of monitoring devices. I was sedated with morphine to control the discomfort and was attended by a technician. In the meantime an internist discussed my condition with Barbara and Janet and felt that the coronary was minor and that my main problem was angina. Apparently, ventricular fibrillation occurred, as determined on the monitor, and the technician was able to inform the specialist directly across the hall. Electrodes were applied to my back, and a few jolts of electricity successfully corrected the fibrillation.

I was fortunate to be in the right place when the crisis occurred. Approximately four minutes after the onset of ventricular fibrillation, permanent brain damage will occur if the condition is not corrected.

During my three weeks in hospital, I asked Janet to bring me as much literature on coronary thrombosis as possible from the library of her hospital. The material was fascinating to digest and included the many predisposing factors as well as advice on the prevention of recurrence. The hospital discharged me with good advice, essentially a repetition of my own research on the subject. A few days after coming home, I received a phone call from my good friend Bill Steinmetz, who was attending a meeting in Chicago. When he learned of my problem, he said, "I am coming to see you," and arrived a few hours later. His visit was much appreciated.

There are many predisposing factors related to coronary thrombosis. A major factor is genetic predisposition. My father died at seventy-three years of age from a massive coronary. My youngest brother died in his early fifties from heart-related problems. My oldest brother required bypass surgery in his early sixties to supply adequate coronary blood flow and died suddenly fifteen years later, according to the coroner, of another heart attack. My only sister has been the victim of two heart attacks that have resulted in severe complicating factors. I had a quadruple bypass when I was sixty-nine, approximately twenty years after my heart attack. All four of my youngest brother Bill's sons have varying degrees of the same genetic problem. A few months after her fiftieth birthday, my daughter experienced angina symptoms. She had a cardiac catheterization to determine whether or not she has the same condition as I have. Fortunately, her arteries were not occluded.

Stress is another major factor that contributes to the problem. There is no doubt in my mind that the dissolution of my professional partnership contributed to my condition. Cigarette smoking (I smoked a pack a day prior to this event) is another of the predisposing factors.

In 1976 I was referred to the Toronto Rehabilitation Centre. This fine organization had developed a comprehensive and successful exercise program for the treatment of people with cardiac problems. Prior to the recommendation of an exercise program, each person is required to undergo a variety of tests to determine the extent of the problem and how vigorous their specific exercise program should be. In my case it was determined that a three-mile walk, completed in forty-five minutes and done five times weekly, would be the appropriate exercise prescription. I carried on this program for several years. Eventually I found that some back problems, caused by disk disease involving the lower three lumbar vertebrae, made walking most uncomfortable.

After recovery I returned to the real-estate business. It became known in my profession that I had started a new career, and calls started to come from veterinarians asking for advice. Within the first year I was involved in the successful sale of a veterinary hospital. The owner of the establishment wished to retire and had no idea as to the value of the premises or the business. My courses on business evaluation helped to establish fair market value for this practice. News of this sale by a satisfied vendor to a satisfied purchaser brought more inquiries. There is no better advertisement for any business than word-of-mouth statements made by happy clients.

I had started to take night courses on various subjects, including appraisal of properties and businesses, as well as the various required courses that would lead to a real-estate broker's license. This preliminary step accomplished, it was time to start my own brokerage and specialize in the evaluation and sale of veterinary practices. I began my company, Multimed Realty, Inc., in 1978 and wound it up in 1991 when Barbara was very ill. We operated the business from our home in a room set aside for the purpose. Barbara played a very important role in the endeavour.

Following graduation in 1975, Janet lived at home for a while. One day she announced that she and Glen were engaged and planned their marriage for May of 1976. While her mother and I had substantial reservations about this decision, we felt that they were adults and we should not interfere. Their marriage took place in our church with a reception at the Scarboro Golf Club following the ceremony. After the reception a lot of the guests came back to our home for some live country and western music provided by friends of mine. All present enjoyed a memorable evening.

When they returned from their honeymoon, they asked us to provide the down payment for a small home they wished to purchase. We agreed, and the purchase was completed. Glen had been a top basketball player at university and continued his affinity for the sport after marriage. Janet had a busy and stressful position as an emergency room nurse. In addition, she had to do most of the housework since Glen was too busy with his basketball activities to be engaged in cooking or cleaning duties. In a short period of time, the marriage started to break down, and they were divorced the following year. Prior to the sale of their home, some renovations were necessary. Even though it was only a few months after the heart attack, I did some of the labour and negotiated with the necessary tradesmen. Fortunately, their marriage produced no children.

Janet moved back to our home and was, as could be expected, very upset about the failed marriage. There was little we could do except provide moral support. Two years later she was offered a position as a nursing instructor in British Columbia. She accepted the offer and spent a year there.

Before going to British Columbia, Janet had applied for admission to various medical colleges. She was aware that passing grades in both organic and inorganic chemistry were needed for admission. She had not taken these subjects during her final year at high school, so she took home studies. It was a rigorous time in her life since she was working full-time. One morning a telephone call came to our home from the dean of medical admissions at McMaster University in Hamilton, requesting her to come for an interview. A successful interview would result in admission to their medical training program. I relayed the call to Janet and, since the date for the interview was within a few days, hoped that she could get the time off for it. This was possible, and she was home in time. Later another call came from the university, stating that she had been accepted. This delighted us all since she had suffered many setbacks since graduating from Queen's.

McMaster required a degree in some other field for eligibility for medical training. Her classmates had earned various degrees, including nursing, law, and degrees in several scientific fields. One classmate had a degree in religion.

Her degree in the nursing field, as well as the experience in emergency medicine, was helpful in understanding the medical courses. McMaster had, and still has, a unique method of teaching medicine in that the students are broken into small study groups, usually five or six students, overseen by the instructor. Each group is given the symptoms of an illness and asked to suggest possible different diagnoses of the condition. This method of study demands use of library facilities to ascertain which of the various possibilities is the most probable diagnosis. McMaster originated this method of teaching, and many medical schools around the world now use it.

During her studies at McMaster, Janet met a young engineer named Michael Tarjan who worked at Dofasco, a large steel-making company in Hamilton. After she graduated they went to Bermuda and were married in 1989. The minister, as well as Janet's cousin Nancy and her husband as the attendants for the bride and groom, were the only ones present at the ceremony. While we were disappointed in not being invited to their very small wedding, we were elated with her choice. Their marriage is very solid and has been blessed with Caroline, my delightful granddaughter, who was born in 1990. She is an outstanding student in both scholastic achievement and athletic ability. Her grandfather is very fond of her.

Following her graduation as physician in 1984, Janet took three years of specialist training in the field of family medicine. Completing this residency, she and a classmate started a practice in Waterdown, Ontario. After a few years in practice, both ladies were asked to go back to McMaster to instruct residents and interns in the field of family medicine. Her partner, Jane, was first to return to teach. Janet followed a few months later. Both enjoyed the challenge of working with doctors in training. To keep up with the young minds, both Janet and Jane found it necessary to keep up to date in their field by constant reading and by attending continuing education meetings.

A disadvantage of their position was the requirement of being on call for emergency duty. If the residents were not able to solve an after-hour problem, they would phone the duty doctor for advice, often in the middle of the night. The duty doctor would often have to return to the office and assist the duty resident. Eventually these hours (as I know from personal experience) become very stressful. Janet is well aware that in all probability she has the genetic defect for cardiac disease. We have often discussed that since I was the victim of a major heart attack at the age of forty-nine, she might be better to return to a private practice. In the fall of 2000, Jane and Janet opened another practice in Waterdown and within a few months had a full complement of patients. Both are interested in providing top quality service and take the necessary time with each patient. The practice is completely computerized; even the prescriptions are printed on the computers.

At the annual meeting of the College of Family Physicians held in Ottawa in October 2000, she was awarded a fellowship in this specialty. Only about 10 percent of family physicians attain this honour. I attended their dinner meeting and was present when various awards were presented. Subsequent to the occasion. I wrote a complimentary letter to her that included a brief review of her life, from childhood to the present. My letter concluded as follows:

> *Your peers in Ottawa have awarded you a distinct honour that, knowing you, will be built upon and never sullied.*
>
> *You know that I am very proud of you for having been such a wonderful daughter and for knowing about your many professional accomplishments. Keep up the good work—first with your family and secondly with your profession. Had she been spared, your mother would have felt the same way. The best way to honour her memory is by continuation of the Barbara Graham Breast Cancer Research Fund. At some point you will have to make the decisions with respect to this project without my assistance.*

There is an old farm expression that states "Every crow thinks that its own egg is the whitest." The reader of this material will recognize that I have feelings similar to the crow.

In 1976 a group of four individuals, including me, formed an investment group. The purpose of the organization was the purchase of a fifty-bed nursing home known to one of the group. The home was devoted to the care of severely handicapped individuals, mostly children, who required more care than their relatives could provide.

Considerable research indicated it to be a good investment. The provincial government paid the fees for the care of the patients. The venture proved successful, and over the next few years we purchased three more small nursing homes, making a total of two hundred beds owned by our company. One of our partners was the managing partner, responsible for the operation of these homes.

Our small group decided to make an investment in the United States and used some of the profits from our nursing home company as well as some additional capital from the partners for the venture. Our first acquisition was a 100-unit apartment building near Tampa, Florida. The municipal regulations in this area allowed the conversion of the units to condominiums. The units sold quickly with a good profit. The next venture was the purchase of a small hotel on St. Petersburg Beach, Florida. The idea behind this purchase was the conversion of the rooms to time-sharing, an idea rapidly gaining popularity. Additional partners were needed to finance this purchase, so a group of twenty-five investors was put together. Within a few months a much larger hotel was for sale, and another group, this time 125 investors, bought it. The goal for the purchase of the larger property was the same: conversion to time-share units.

Some of us had apprehensions about the rapid expansion and concern about the concept of time-share units; really, we had no understanding of it. This concern was exacerbated when the driving force behind the two groups, a real-estate broker from Ontario, was chosen to be the general manager of both operations as well as chief of sales for the time-share units. Some of us objected to this dual role, and he was removed from the position of general manager for the smaller building. Our attempt to remove him from the larger building failed, since he had a group of loyal followers. The rumour was circulated that this individual had contravened the regulations of the Ontario Securities Commission in that, in contradiction of the rules, he had not filed a prospectus for the venture. Within a few days an offer was made to the dissenters to purchase their shares at cost. Certain that the venture of the larger property would fail under his management, we accepted. This turned out to be the case, and the loyal followers lost all of their investment.

Is there a lesson to be learned from this experience? "Avoid involvement in a venture that you do not understand."

The managing partner of the nursing homes decided that he would like to purchase all of the shares of the other three partners. He offered his shares of the Florida ventures as well as some additional funds to complete the transaction. This seemed to be a fair deal to all, and it was completed.

These time-share ventures were not productive, but we did not lose any capital. One of my reasons for wanting to invest outside Canada was my feeling that our country was losing ground in industrial productivity because of the giveaway policies of our federal government. Predictably, unfortunate things would happen, such as increasing national debt and decline in the value of our currency. We decided to continue investing in the USA as opportunities arose.

For tax purposes, as the result of good legal and accounting advice, a Barbara and I formed a Canadian company with a subsidiary U.S. company one hundred percent owned by the Canadian company. Any real estate investments in the USA are owned by the subsidiary company. Since the beginning, further real estate investments have been added and involvement with others no longer occurs, except for a land development venture in Bradenton, Florida. This investment has now come to fruition and has been profitable.

When the veterinary partnership broke apart, a company called Pet Care Limited, formed when the practice started in

1957, owned the real estate occupied by the Amherst Veterinary Hospital. Dick and I and our wives owned the shares. Rent was paid by the professional practice to the company. This served as a tax advantage since the tax rate was lower on the company than it was on the income of the practitioners. The dissolution of the partnership did not include the real estate, and Barbara and I remained part owners of the real estate through the company. A new lease was drawn between the new partnership and the company. It called for a fixed amount of rent for a five-year period with options to renew for two further five-year periods. It was a net-net lease, meaning that the tenant was responsible for all expenses pertaining to the premises. The lease described the property that included the building and all of the land owned by the company. It also included the provision that if this agreement on rental value of renewals was not accepted and the new rental amount was not agreed upon, each side would have an appraisal as to fair market value. If there was no agreement an arbitrator would be chosen, and his decision would be binding on all parties. Similar arrangements were the case with the secondary practice in Oshawa except that in this case the shareholders of the real estate were the four veterinarians and their wives.

When the first five-year period elapsed, notification was received that the option to renew was being exercised. Since I was now in the business of the evaluation and sale of veterinary premises, I was well aware of current market rates. My rate was unacceptable to the tenants, so each side appointed an appraiser. There was considerable disparity in the two opinions, mostly due to the fact that the tenant's appraisal stated that not all of the land was necessary for the operation of the practice. When it came to arbitration, the arbitrator wrote that the lease document clearly stated that all of the land was included and that the tenant's appraiser should have been aware of this. After the next five-year period, disagreement again occurred. After arbitration, my evaluation, similar to opinion of the expert I employed, was accepted.

Multimed Realty, Inc. kept me busy but was much less stressful than my former career had been. My working area was essentially in Ontario, except for a few transactions out of province. In time more people asked for written evaluations of the value of the business aspects of their practices. There were two main reasons for these opinions of value. Often a practice was taking in a new partner or the senior partners were retiring and wanted to establish a figure fair to all. The next most common reason for such an opinion related to marital dissolution. Because of the Family Law Act in Ontario, at dissolution each spouse was entitled to 50 percent of the fair market value of appreciated value of acquired assets during the years of marriage. In most cases a husband owned the practice and hired me to prepare an Opinion of Value. In two cases the veterinarian was a female needing advice. In both of these cases I did not feel that the husband of the veterinarian should have benefited from the law, as neither of these men had been of much help to his professional wife. However, the law prevailed. If there were any disagreement with my opinion, the other side would get another opinion, often prepared by an accountant.

One such case aroused my interest, since the opposing lawyers disagreed. The case went to court. When I was called to the witness stand, the lawyer for the wife started to ask me questions related to my expertise in the subject. He first asked whether I had an accounting degree, to which I replied in the negative. He then asked whether or not I had an MBA. Again I replied that I did not have such a degree. The judge then asked me how many sales of veterinary hospitals I had made and how many Opinions of Value I had written. At that time the combined number of sales and written evaluations was approximately two hundred. The judge then said that because of that much experience he would consider me to be an expert witness on this subject. When the chartered accountant who had done the evaluation for the wife was called to the stand, the lawyer for the husband asked him how many evaluations he had done on veterinary practices. The answer was, "This is the first one that I have done." The main reason that his evaluation was so much higher than mine was that accounting firms have a much higher margin of profit than do veterinary hospitals and this had been factored into his figures. The judge accepted my opinion as being the most realistic.

Small businesses, including veterinary practices, are no different from large corporations in that they are subject to loss of income when employees are dishonest. The following anecdote illustrates such a case.

Dr. Bert Barrett immigrated to Canada from South Africa where he had owned and operated veterinary practices. For some time he was employed in an Ontario veterinary practice to get experience with the problems animals experience in his adopted country. Ready to go on his own, he phoned me to see whether any practices were for sale meeting his criteria. I had just listed for sale a large dog-and-cat boarding kennel. This facility had been in operation for a long time, had a good cash flow, and could readily support the purchase price of the property and the business. Bert and I reasoned that with the large number of dogs and cats passing through the facility, veterinary clients would be attracted to a practice at the same location. There was adequate room in the building for a veterinary office. The purchase was completed, and the renovations resulted in an attractive facility.

Shortly after Bert's new business was started, a small veterinary clinic located about five miles from Bert's office was listed for sale with my company. Bert and I felt that he could operate both practices, since his own practice was still in its growth phase. A few months after the purchase of the new practice, which was in a leased building, the owner of the building approached us to see if we would be interested in buying the building. The price as determined by its owner was realistic, so Bert and I purchased it as partners.

Bert employed a non-professional assistant at his primary practice. As well as looking after animals, the assistant was responsible for the banking of both practices. After a period of time the ratio of income to expenses showed a substantial reduction. Obviously something was very wrong. We asked for the assistance of the Toronto Police Department Fraud Squad. They gave up on the case, saying that it was unlikely to make any charges stick since other staff as well as the suspect had access to the invoices. We decided to do a personal investigation. This meant going over all of the patient files and financial records.

With each client transaction a duplicate numbered financial slip was made out, one going to the client as a receipt and the other retained by the practice. This number was typed on the medical chart of the patient. One weekend I took all of the slips as well as the medical charts of the new clinic to my home and compared the slips with the medical charts. After comparing many slips and charts, I found that approximately 10 percent of the slips were missing. It was simple to determine how much money was missing since the medical charts had the amount that the client had been charged on each visit as well as on the slips.

At the same time Bert and his wife Sue did a similar investigation at the boarding kennel and its associated veterinary clinic. Appointment calendars and the boarding reservation books were examined.

The investigation completed, Bert confronted the employee with the evidence. Soon after this conversation the employee tried to burn the slips, but we recovered many, still readable. Bert and I met with the employee and made him aware that he could be imprisoned. This terrified him, and he offered to sign a promissory note to repay the total amount. He would not have managed it without the help of his wife. She was outraged to learn that he had stolen from us and vowed to pay it back. We went to a lawyer who had been a prosecuting crown attorney and had him draw up an appropriate agreement. The employee agreed to repay the embezzled amount of more than $20,000.00.

Repayment of the total amount took three years. To make this restitution, his wife took a job and he found another position. Good records had allowed the amateur detectives to prove the theft.

After the renovation of the new clinic and by a substantial increase in client numbers, the real estate and practice were sold with appreciation in value. Bert's practice in the kennel operation had grown to the point that it occupied all of his time and required the employment of another veterinarian. Bert and his wife Sue have raised four children, all university graduates. I like to think of Bert as the type of new Canadian needed in Canada. He and Sue have made a great contribution to the country.

Letters to Politicians

Introduction

Twice during my years of practice I was approached to consider running as a candidate for the Progressive Conservative Party, once as a federal and once as a provincial candidate. The requests came from high in the party, and I was assured that in all probability I would be successful. I declined both invitations. I would be required to vote on party lines as opposed to, as a member of either Parliament, being able to make my own decision as to what was best for the people of my riding as well as for our province and for Canada.

Ambrose Bierce, the American post-Civil-War writer, wrote: "Lifelong exposure to the hypocrisies of politics leaves curmudgeons united in their disdain of politicians of all stripes." The *New Lexicon Webster's Encyclopaedic Dictionary* defines "curmudgeon" as "a bad-tempered, churlish man." In his *Devil's Dictionary* Bierce defined a conservative as "a statesman who is enamoured of existing evils as distinguished from a liberal who wishes to replace them with others." Since at last count in Canada we now have four major political parties, it is reasonable to consider that there could be even more duplicity in Canadian government. By Bierce's definition, I guess I am a curmudgeon!

Both before and after my active days in practice, I wrote many letters to politicians, usually complaining about government waste. While I usually received replies to my letters, my complaints seem to have done little to improve the problems.

Chapter Twenty-Nine

Search and Rescue

In late 1972 a bush plane was on a rescue mission in north-western Canada to transport an extremely ill child as well as the child's mother and a nurse skilled in emergency care. The plane, piloted by its owner, a Mr. Hartwell, crashed before it got to the hospital. Two of the passengers were killed in the crash. In spite of an extensive search by aircraft of the Armed Forces, the plane could not be found for more than a month. Eventually it was located by another bush pilot, a friend of Mr. Hartwell.

Following the rescue of the two survivors, it was learned that to avoid starvation they had consumed some of the flesh of the deceased. The account of their ordeal was front-page news for some time.

The newspapers alleged that restraints in the defense budget resulted in the search being ineffective. Now, more than thirty years later, we still have under-funded armed services.

I was of the opinion it should be mandatory that every aircraft be equipped with emergency electronic locator transmitters so that a search aircraft could readily find a crashed airplane. On December 14, 1972, I wrote, in part, to Dr. Reginald Stackhouse, MP for Scarborough East:

> *It has been estimated that this search will cost the Canadian taxpayer 1.7 million dollars. As a taxpayer I believe I have a right to insist on some basic fundamentals. These fundamentals should include at least the following:*
>
> *– Efficient S.A.R. aircraft and personnel*
>
> *– Mandatory electronic locator transmitter on all aircraft*
>
> *– Mandatory instrument flying certification for all pilots*
>
> *– Chartered private pilots from the crash area to augment SAR*
>
> *– Stringently enforced DOT regulations*

As well as from Dr. Stackhouse, I received acknowledgement from the Office of the Minister for National Defence and from Robert Stanfield, Leader of the Opposition.

By an act in Parliament a few months later it became a law that all aircraft be required to have the locator transmitter. I like to think that my letter to Dr. Stackhouse had a bearing on the enactment of this new legislation.

Chapter Thirty

Parliamentary Pay Raise

In 1981, parliamentarians voted themselves a handsome pay raise. The new representative for my riding, Scarborough East, The Honourable Mr. Gordon Gilchrist, voted against the measure and announced that he would refuse the salary increase. This prompted me to write, in part:

> *It seems to me that you are one of a very few representatives of the people of Canada who is more concerned with the state of the economy than of his own personal welfare. I compliment you on your lonely and courageous stand on July 9 as well as for your refusal to take the unjustified salary increase. Can the people of Canada really be expected to bite the bullet when parliamentarians and civil servants treat themselves so beneficially with respect to salaries and indexed pensions?*
>
> *By and large Canadians are getting extremely poor value for the money spent on government. Members of*

Parliament like to compare themselves to executives in the private sector. I feel quite sure that you, as a businessman, would agree with my contention that few of the 282 Members would have a position for very long if their salaries were paid directly by industry. Industry simply wouldn't tolerate executives having the level of financial incompetence displayed by many members in Ottawa.

The lifeblood of an economy is its productivity. The insidious legacy perpetuated on Canadians by governments, particularly for the last twenty years, is the philosophy that a citizen does not have to produce a day's work for a day's pay. It is reasonable to assume that politicians for the most part consider that a vote bought with taxpayer's money is an easier vote to obtain than a vote earned by good government. It seems to me that the recent budget was designed with this philosophy in mind. Hopefully it will backfire on its architect.

The automobile industry, as well as many Canadian industries, is in difficulty because of lack of worker productivity and because of poor planning by management and government. Wouldn't it be reasonable to emulate the Japanese and to put their efficiency to work in Canada rather than simply to restrict their imports?

Japan has few natural resources except for its people and its leaders, who have worked together to bring the country from economic disaster to world eminence. It is ironical that Canada has abundant natural resources, no leadership to speak of, and a work force educated to the philosophy hereinbefore described. Does Canada have to file bankruptcy before a turning point towards economic recovery can be reached?

Yesterday's separatist win in Alberta may well be as significant as the initial Quebec separatist seats in that provincial legislature. At best, the Alberta development is a sign of deep discontent with the management of this country.

Until representatives of the people of Canada put political expediency and personal greed behind, I can see little change except for a worsening of the economy as well as other problems such as a permanent division of the country. It is all very well to hope that an improvement of the American economy will pull ours up—is this all that we have the right to expect?

Yours sincerely,
J.E.B. Graham, D.V.M.

P.S. Enclosed please find a copy of my formula for parliamentary reform. Feel free to circulate it to your 281 colleagues who are far more in need of criticism than are you.

The "formula" referred to was in the form of a satirical letter sent to various federal politicians to exhibit some of my frustrations. *Webster's Dictionary* defines *satire* as "the use of ridicule, sarcasm, irony, etc., to expose, attack or deride vices, follies, etc." While my letter was intended to be humourous, I felt that most of it did apply to politicians:

On February 3, 1982, MP Gordon Taylor, referring to Mr. Trudeau, said that $656.25 was too much rent to pay for a turkey and was promptly cut off by the Speaker. Perhaps the reason Mr. Taylor was cut off was that to some degree the remark was inaccurate. Everyone knows that a turkey is a pompous bird with poor powers of flight. The Speaker knows, as does the Canadian taxpayer, that Mr. Trudeau is pompous but often flies long distances. As a matter of fact, most cabinet ministers should not be called turkeys for the same reason.

Sow's Ear to Silk Purse

Over the years I have heard the names of many animals used in comparison to politicians. As a veterinarian I feel qualified to comment that most of these analogies are unfair to the animals concerned.

I have heard politicians referred to as tomcats. A tomcat marks off a specific area, to protect his territory from other invading tomcats and to screw anything he can in his area. While politicians, especially finance ministers, certainly screw every possible taxpayer, they don't mark off specific boundaries. Finance ministers consider the whole area, whether federal or provincial as the case may be, to be their own territory and for this reason disregard smaller definitive boundaries. One would therefore have to assume that politicians are more insatiable than tomcats, and that is hard to imagine. When one considers the fighting part associated with territorial marking, the analogy is accurate, as evidenced by federal-provincial bickering with respect to some aspects of taxation.

Politicians are often referred to as sheep. A sheep is a stupid animal that blindly follows the leader, even into the slaughter pen. While this comparison has some validity, one has to consider, in fairness to the sheep, another aspect of the matter. A sheep is a very useful creature in that it produces meat and wool, while politicians rarely produce anything useful. I submit that to call politicians "sheep" is an insult to the ovine species.

How about the comparison of politicians to ostriches? It certainly can be conceded that like ostriches, politicians often bury their heads in the sand and frequently lay large eggs. Ostriches, however, are useful in that they produce valuable feathers.

I have heard politicians referred to as "dogs." There are more than 120 breeds of dogs, most of which have some degree of usefulness. For this reason, as with sheep and ostriches, it is not right to call politicians "dogs." It would however be fair to say that dogs act like tomcats on occasion, so there is partial justification in the terminology.

Parrots are large birds that often speak by imitating what they hear around them. In addition, they often inflict severe bites on an unwary victim. Most parrots lay small eggs. Politicians could qualify in certain respects when compared to parrots in that they rarely have anything original to say and that they frequently bite the taxpayer inflicting severe wounds. It must be considered, however, that the taxpayer can hardly be considered unwary in this day and age. In addition, the eggs laid by politicians are normally large rather than small.

While at first consideration the comparison of politicians and jackasses seems appropriate, I take particular exception to this analogy. A jackass is a small stubborn animal, usually closely attached to his master. He works very hard bearing heavy loads and asks for nothing in return except for a bit to eat and a little water. While politicians are stubborn and closely attached to their master, the taxpayer, their wants tend to eclipse those of the loyal jackass. Whoever heard of a jackass bleeding his master dry by means of an indexed pension?

A bull is an animal that produces excrement with a common name. While it is fair to say that this name aptly describes much political rhetoric, other comparisons of politicians to male bovines should be discouraged. It must be remembered that bulls produce meat, hides, and offspring and therefore are producers of useful commodities. Furthermore, when they sire offspring, accurate records are normally kept. Severe penalties are imposed for falsification of documents. These standards are not always adhered to with respect to the offspring of politicians.

The term "sly as a fox" is often used in reference to politicians. The fox is a very devious animal that sneaks up on its prey without the victim being aware of impending doom. While politicians, often deservedly, have the reputation of being devious, they are usually less intelligent than the fox in that the taxpayer is becoming increasingly aware of his impending doom.

Chicken is another name sometimes used in reference to politicians. When confined to small spaces chickens often peck the heads of each other causing moderate to severe damage. This type of cannibalism is often seen in the House of Commons debates and in leadership infighting. Chickens are easily intimidated much as are backbench politicians. The comparison breaks down when the question of productivity is considered.

The observer of pigs would be quick to point out that pigs do not normally defecate in their own nest and are very greedy individuals. A similarity can be demonstrated when one compares pigs to politicians, except for the use of their nest.

It is the considered opinion of this writer that while all the above animal species can be compared to politicians, all fail when the element of productivity is considered. A better analogy would be to compare politicians to various species of the monkey family. Most members of this large group of animals, like the Liberals, exhibit socialist tendencies.

Since, as herein before described, all of the animals considered have more utility than parliamentarians, I therefore recommend that a comparable species such as the monkey or the ape replace the 282 Members of Parliament. Each animal would be given a yes–no button to be pushed when a vote is to be taken in the House. This new parliament should be better than what we have for the following reasons:

1. Any vote taken could be decided by intelligence rather than by following party lines.

2. The chance of a correct decision on any problem would be 50-50 even if an ape of low intelligence had been sent to Ottawa.
3. Since apes detest pigs, pork barrel politics would be eliminated.

There were few replies from the politicians who received a copy of my comments. However, I did receive this in a reply from Mr. Gordon Gilchrist, Conservative member from my riding. I should point out that the Conservatives were in the Official Opposition at the time:

I hope you will continue to make your views known but, with great respect, I suggest you leave the Official Opposition members out of your barnyard scenario until we have earned membership through poor performance, something which we have not been permitted to do by a public which has preferred deceit and acrimony to substantive policy.

Despite government changes since this was written, my opinion of the Canadian political system has not changed. All political parties pander to the voters through inducements to attract support. What would be wrong with saying "We have only so much funding, and we wish to spread it for the benefit of all Canadians"? They could also say "We will not use the dissemination of taxpayer's money to buy the votes of vested interests."

Chapter Thirty-One

Poaching

The April 4, 1988, CBC television program "The Journal" was substantially devoted to allegations of extensive poaching of game animals such as caribou, elk, bear, and deer. The program indicated that animal parts such as penises, testicles, gallbladders, and antlers are very desirable in the oriental pharmaceutical industry. The films showed truckloads of antlers, many of which had come from Canada, being shipped from United States ports. The program explained that Canadian conservation officers experience great difficulty with their attempts to control the problem.

This was the opening paragraph of a letter I wrote to the Honourable Vincent Kerrio, Minister of Natural Resources. I continued:

Antlers are apparently more valuable to the oriental pharmaceutical industry if the rack is in velvet. Since the velvet is usually rubbed off prior to the hunting season, it would appear that many of these animals are killed during the summer months, with obvious waste of meat. The television report indicated that bears are shot with often only the gallbladder retrieved. This would suggest a similar wastage of meat.

I am a veterinarian and an outdoorsman. It is my opinion as a veterinarian that any medical benefits to be derived from the use of such animal parts is open to question. Apparently it is commonly believed that some of these parts, when consumed, possess potent aphrodisiac properties. Even if this could be proven accurate, I do not subscribe to the illegal, wholesale slaughter of animals in order that some affluent, aging men may be provided with sexual activity beyond their capability.

A few months ago, the federal government put up some trial balloons with respect to projected tough measures in dealing with the illicit narcotics trade. As I recall, these measures included, upon conviction, increased fines and jail terms. Additionally, and of considerable importance, suggested measures included confiscation of funds obtained illegally from the drug trade and also of equipment such as airplanes, boats and cars. I would recommend that your Ministry give consideration to similar measures. I am aware that your present legislation provides for seizure and sale of equipment. How often is this applied? It is reasonable to assume that a poacher might have second thoughts about his activity if there was a real chance that his airplane worth $100,000.00 or his vehicle worth $25,000.00 could be confiscated as part of the penalty.

Very seldom does a political issue arise where the only dissenters would be lawbreakers. Voting Canadians, except for those profiting from illegal activity, whether or not they approve of legitimate hunting, would almost unanimously approve your strong intervention. The political benefit should be obvious. Politicians of 1988 need some issues with little political risk.

This letter was widely circulated and I received a sizeable volume of response. Mr. Kerrio replied, in part:

I am concerned, as you are, that Ontario's wildlife should not be placed in jeopardy by illegal commercial poaching. Poaching is certainly a potentially serious problem in this province. However, I do not believe that the actual problem in Ontario is nearly as serious as "The Journal" made it seem.

Ontario's Conservation Officers, who are out in the field every day, have a good feel for the amount of illegal activity that is occurring and they believe the situation is well under control. Nevertheless, I trust you will be pleased to hear that proposed amendments to the Game and Fish Act would increase the maximum fine for commercial violations from $5,000 to $50,000 and permit the court to impose jail sentences...

Yours sincerely,

Vincent G. Kerrio
Minister

Chapter Thirty-Two

Gun Control and Immigration

Canadians are well aware that legislation on gun control has been introduced. As often happens with many new regulations, the cost of this legislation to date far exceeds the original estimates. Major mistakes such as computer problems have contributed to the confusion. Considerable opposition by farmers, sportsmen and aboriginal groups is evident. The legislation fails to address most of the problems I raised in a letter to the prime minister, the immigration minister, and the minister of justice, specifically that the criminal element responsible for most of the gun related deaths is not the major thrust of the legislation. Several provinces have indicated that they will not enforce this law and any charges for failing to comply will have to be laid by the federal government. The text of this letter follows:

June 23, 1994

The Right Honourable Jean Chrétien
Prime Minister of Canada
The Honourable Sergio Marchi
Immigration Minister
The Honourable Allan Rock
Minister of Justice

Gentlemen;

Re: Gun Control Legislation and Immigration
Legislation

Since legislation in these areas is due for review and
revision, I would like to address both in this letter. The
Metropolitan Toronto Police Department, as well as
other police departments, have an oath to serve and protect the public. I would hope that the House of Commons
of Canada could consider adopting such an undertaking. It would be fair to say that previous and present
governments have been remiss in protecting the public
from undesirable immigrants.

Mr. Chrétien has publicly stated that better legislation with respect to gun control is forthcoming. Let us
hope that the new legislation is in fact better. All
Canadians would agree that senseless slaughter of
humans must be controlled. This cannot be done by
focusing primarily on legitimate sportsmen. Present legislation requires that legitimate purchasers of firearms
have acquisition certificates and proper gun storage in
locked cabinets or by special trigger locks. Legal handgun owners are tightly regulated. An idea being proposed would require warehousing of sporting weapons
in some type of government controlled storage facilities
which would be located away from cities. Legislators

proposing such a preposterous idea should be aware that armories and police stations have, in the past, been burglarized and weapons stolen. If government and police stations cannot protect their own firearms, how can they protect the firearms of the legitimate sportsman? My guess is that criminals would be delighted to have vast numbers of weapons in one place and would devise ways to steal these weapons.

Most crimes involving the use of guns are not committed by legitimate sportsman or by their weapons. Most crimes involving guns are committed by criminals using handguns which have been smuggled into Canada. The Ontario government is currently considering a bill with respect to ammunition control. While this may have a minor benefit, ammunition could, like handguns, be smuggled from the USA or from other provinces.

Recently I delivered to a local police station, for destruction, a legal handgun that I have owned for some thirty years and for which I have no further use. At present I own, for sporting purposes, three rifles and one shotgun. I have no objection to these guns being registered if such legislation is passed. I do object to the enactment of laws which do not address the primary problem.

The primary problem that must be addressed is control of criminals who use illegal weapons—not the legitimate sportsman. I propose the following:

1. Simple possession of an illegal weapon should be punished by a substantial sentence—at least five years in penitentiary with no chance of parole. If such an illegal weapon is used in the commission of a crime, there should be a minimum sentence of ten years with no chance of parole, in addition to whatever penalty is required for the crime itself. If a person is killed during the commission of a crime, I would further propose either capital punishment for the criminal or some number of strokes of the lash followed by imprisonment for life with no parole. Many bleeding hearts will say that this is cruel and unusual punishment. If such penalties were well known, I am sure that the dregs of society who commit such crimes would be more reluctant to prey on those who are unable to defend themselves.

2. *Plea bargaining of firearms related charges should be eliminated; current laws are emasculated by plea bargaining.*

3. *Military assault type weapons are of no use to a sportsman and should be banned.*

4. *The firepower of weapons in the hands of criminals usually exceeds that of police officers. Funds should be available to upgrade the service revolvers of policemen.*

5. *Any individual who has a criminal record in his own country should be refused admission to Canada.*

6. *Parliament should submit to all Canadians a referendum, binding upon the House of Commons, asking for the return of capital punishment under certain circumstances such as the murder of a policeman. There is no doubt in my mind that most Canadians would support such a referendum.*

Chapter Thirty-Three

Immigration Legislation

Canadian citizenship should be conditional upon good behaviour. Such legislative change would provide that within some period of time following arrival in Canada—say ten years—an immigrant convicted of a serious crime would be deported with no recourse. Canada's immigration and refugee policies are the most generous in the world. Canada's accumulated deficit is one of the worst in the world. One does not have to be a rocket scientist to realize that Canada cannot afford this open door policy which must add billions to our overwhelming deficit.

From Confederation until the last twenty or twenty-five years, Canada's immigration system was essentially based on the point system. In other words, the acceptance of new Canadians was based on what they could do for the country. Now the highest percentage of immigrants comes in as family class (related to someone liv-

ing in Canada) or as refugees. In many cases these individuals are unable to contribute to Canada's economy because of lack of skills or inability to converse in English or French and become a burden on the welfare system and on the medical system.

Most Canadians agree that we need more immigrants. It seems to me that more emphasis must be placed on selection of immigrants who will add to, rather than detract from, Canada's economy. Now that we are in the information (computer) age, let us compile information on immigrants from various countries. Such information would likely demonstrate that immigrants from some countries are more likely to be useful citizens while immigrants from other countries are more likely to overload our welfare system or to become involved in criminal activities because they lack the skills to compete in the workforce.

In addition to screening potential immigrants for their ability to contribute to rather than to detract from Canada's economy, all candidates should be screened for various diseases. I really can't see why we should burden our health-care system by admitting known carriers of AIDS, tuberculosis, etc.

Recently in Toronto, Oniel Rohan Grant was charged in the Just Desserts slaying of Georgina Leimonis. Prior to this murder Grant was ordered to be deported for various crimes including weapons offences. This deportation order was overruled by a gullible woman representing the Immigration and Refugee Board. She believed the story that he was going to change his ways! Why should any individual have the power to overrule a deportation order?

Yesterday Constable Bayliss was buried. His murderer, Clinton Gayle, was ordered deported three years ago, but his file was mysteriously misplaced. How will you, Mr. Marchi, punish such stupidity? The front page of today's Toronto Star *quotes Mr. Marchi as stating that*

Gayle is as much a product of the Canadian society as of the country where he was born. What are you trying to do, Mr. Marchi? Perhaps it is an attempt to take the heat off the Department of Immigration.

Sooner or later some Canadian will lay a charge of criminal negligence because of lack of care in enforcing deportation orders. I wonder who will be charged—the culpable woman in the Grant case, the incompetent civil servants in the Gayle case, or perhaps past or present ministers responsible in the cases?

According to today's Globe and Mail, one Alan Lennon of the Immigration Union stated in reference to people living illegally in Canada: "If you keep your head down and no one turns you in, we aren't going to come and get you." According to the same article, there are 26,000 unexecuted deportation orders. Mr. Marchi, how many more young policemen have to be killed before you live up to your responsibility? Priority must be given to getting these undesirables out of Canada.

Several years ago a man named Ng was incarcerated in Calgary for about five years. This man had been convicted in California on charges that he had murdered some eleven people. Canada resisted his extradition to California on the grounds that he might be executed if he were returned to California. What right has Canada to interfere with the judicial system of another country? Deportation was finally allowed after we had spent several hundred thousand dollars of taxpayers' money on his incarceration and on his legal appeals. What a hell of a waste of taxpayers' money!

Gentlemen, your legislation needs revision. I hope that you will find my comments of use in your deliberations.

Yours very truly,
J. B. Graham D.V.M.

Copies to: Doering, Charles, C.F.R.B. Toronto
Downing, John, Editor, The Toronto Sun
Francis, Diane, Editor, The Financial Post
Harris, Mike, Leader, Ontario Progressive Conservative Party
Honderich, John, Editor, The Toronto Star
Manning, Preston, Leader, Reform Party of Canada
McCormack, William, Police Chief, Metropolitan Toronto
Morgan, Rick, V. P., Ontario Federation of Anglers & Hunters
Myers, Burton, Editor, Ontario Out of Doors
Peters, Douglas, MP, Scarborough East
Rae, Bob, Premier Ontario
Thorsell, William, Editor in Chief, The Globe & Mail
Others, friends and acquaintances whom I will encourage to support my views.

The editor of *The Financial Post* and the staff inspector of the Metropolitan Toronto Police sent letters of appreciation, as did several professional colleagues. The letter generated a great volume of response, not just to me but between government offices. Highlights are included.

Mr. John Nunziata, MP for York South-Weston, wrote to me, in part:

> *With respect to the immigration system in Canada, I too feel that the bureaucratic bungling that allowed Mr. Gayle to remain in Canada for two years after he was ordered deported is unacceptable. For this reason...I suggested that a special police unit be established to ensure that convicted criminals with deportation orders be immediately located and escorted out of Canada.*
>
> *On July 8, 1994, my colleague Sergio Marchi, the Minister of Immigration, announced a comprehensive*

reform of Canada's removal policies including the creation of a special Immigration RCMP task force to crack down on foreign criminals. Clearly, such immediate action against individuals such as Oneil Grant and Clinton Gayle would have prevented recent tragedies.

The Township of Dawn passed a resolution:

Dear Mr. Graham:

Re: Gun Control Legislation and Immigration Legislation
As per our phone conversation of this afternoon, Council reviewed your letter on the above matter at a recent meeting. A resolution was passed supporting your letter and notification of this action is being forwarded to the various members of Parliament and provincial legislature.

This resolution went to the top:

Office of the Prime Minister
Ottawa, Canada MA 0A2
September 22, 1994

Dear Ms. MacDougal,
On behalf of the Right Honourable Jean Chrétien, I wish to acknowledge receipt of your correspondence of August 23 regarding Council's support of a letter by J.E.B. Graham on gun control and immigration legislation. Thank you for writing the Prime Minister. You may be assured that your comments have been carefully noted.

Yours sincerely,
Jennifer Holmes
Assistant - Correspondence

Sow's Ear to Silk Purse

On October 4, 1994, Mr. Allan Rock, Minister of Justice, responded to the Township of Dawn:

On behalf of the Honourable Sergio Marchi, Minister of Citizenship and Immigration, I want to thank you for your letter of August 23, 1994, and enclosure concerning gun control and immigration legislation. The Minister has requested that I respond to your concerns.

On the subject of gun control, the Prime Minister, in his remarks during the election campaign, indicated the government's concern about violent crime. Canadians have a right to expect their government to take appropriate action in this area. This will include legislation dealing with firearms and other weapons. In this regard, difficult decisions will have to be made...

My colleagues and I have also begun to examine the difficult problems of firearm smuggling and theft from legal owners. Strict legislation must be enforced, and part of that enforcement must be dedicated to ensuring that access and the registration controls which apply to law-abiding and responsible firearm owners are not simply evaded by others.

I believe in strong and effective gun control measures, and I am committed to taking effective steps to reduce violent crime and improve public safety in Canada, but I appreciate that the interests of all Canadians must be taken into account in developing and implementing criminal justice policies.

Our commitment is to strict legislation, but I assure you that we will also be fair in developing and implementing firearms control policies. The legitimate concerns of farmers, hunters, and subsistence hunters will be respected and we shall make every attempt to minimize any inconvenience to these users.

I appreciate having had your views regarding this important issue brought to my attention.

Yours very truly,
Allan Rock

On September 9, 1994, the same Minister of Justice wrote to me, in part:

While I recognize that many Canadians own and use firearms prudently and responsibly, the presence of firearms under any circumstances carries with it a risk for the safety of all of us, and I am convinced that more can and must be done. Over the coming months, my colleagues and I will be reviewing options in this area, and I assure you that no option will be excluded from our review if it offers a reasonable prospect of addressing concerns about violence in any area of our society.

In a letter to me dated September 13, 1994, Mr. Mousaw of Citizenship and Immigration made a number of points. One was that criminals should not be permitted to abuse our immigration process. He adds that the Minister has made it a priority to restore confidence in the system:

Over the past few months, Minister Marchi has made it a priority to restore public confidence in the immigration and refugee programs. In keeping with this position, on June 17, 1994, the Minister announced amendments to the Immigration Act to deal with abuse and fraud, including steps to stop the smuggling of travel documents through international mail. He introduced measures that address abuse of the refugee determination system by criminals, improve the operation of the Immigration and Refugee Board and streamline its appeals process.

Subsequently, on July 7, 1994, a comprehensive reorientation of Canada's removals policy was announced, based on the following three elements:
1. The new removals strategy will concentrate first and foremost on getting criminals out of this country.

2. *A special task force, including twenty police officers on assignment from the RCMP, has been established to concentrate immediately and exclusively on tracking and removing foreign criminals with serious convictions who have evaded removal action. Our immigration officers will be on the task force, which will also be supported by local police forces. Moreover, ten additional immigration staff will be assigned to support the task force in the greater Toronto area. As well, the complement of thirty-six immigration investigators in Toronto will be maintained.*

3. *The cases of refused refugee claimants who have not been removed in the past because of civil unrest in their homeland will be resolved. We will ensure that deferred removals are acted upon efficiently and fairly.*

Nine years later it seems that the problem has worsened. None of the elements listed by Mr. Mousaw has been successfully implemented. When the Metro Toronto Police Chief requested access to the list of some 30,000 people under deportation orders, he was refused, and the government cited the privacy rights of these people as an excuse. The reprint from the *National Post* cites the probability of 10,000 terrorists living in Canada. Surely allowing these people to stay in Canada should not be a priority of our Government. I quote him: "I want to stress that these changes and improvements are consistent with the government's commitment to deal firmly with the abuse of Canada's immigration and refugee programs." So much for the protestations on making things better! It would be fair to say that our problems with immigrants have worsened rather than improved since my letter of 1994.

Chapter Thirty-Four

To the Honourable
Paul Martin

At the time of writing and editing (early 2004), The Honourable Paul Martin has become prime minister of Canada. A decade ago I wrote the following to Mr. Martin in his (then) new capacity as Minister of Finance:

November 7, 1994
The Honourable Paul Martin
Minister of Finance
Parliament Buildings
Ottawa, Ontario

Dear Sir,
First let me congratulate you on your determination to reduce the deficit and ultimately reduce the national debt. You have stated that the national debt is a millstone around the neck of Canada and must be corrected. If we cannot solve our own financial mess, in time the

International Monetary Fund will be called upon to correct our problems. Their medicine would be very harsh. Many former Ministers of Finance have discussed deficit reduction but in fact have allowed the deficits to escalate. You may be our last Minister of Finance with the power to improve our fiscal malaise.

You have asked Canadians for advice as to how best to accomplish deficit reduction. This letter with its suggestions for your consideration has been written by a senior citizen of Canada who is greatly concerned with the economic future of our country.

The Globe and Mail *on November 1, 1994, published a large advertisement by the National Citizens Coalition stating where Canadian MPs stand on their Gold Plated Pension Plan. I note with interest that only 13 Liberal MPs showed support for major pension reform. You, as well as Mr. Chrétien, Mr. Marchi, Mr. Peters, Mr. Rock, Mr. Axworthy, and other Cabinet Ministers failed to answer the request for their position on the issue. Surprisingly, Mr. Manning failed to answer as well; not surprisingly Mr. Bouchard also failed to respond. Presumably by their lack of response those failing to respond agree that they are entitled to these munificent pensions which to say the least are not acceptable to the Canadian taxpayer.*

Mr. Bouchard has stated that if he is successful in pulling Quebec out of Canada, he as well as any other Bloc Quebecois member with six years in the House of Commons will still be entitled to life pensions from Canada. Legislation should be introduced immediately to thwart Mr. Bouchard's pension ambitions.

I suggest, Mr. Martin, that if you are going to sell austerity to Canadians in your next budget, you should show by example and change the pension plans of politicians and bureaucrats to correspond with those plans available to the private sector.

To the Honourable Paul Martin

Patronage:

The cost of patronage to the taxpayer must be addressed. What is wrong with the appointment of someone qualified to fill a job rather than to appoint some political hack or party supporter to fill the same position? I view with distaste the appointment of political "has-beens" to offices in which they have no experience while at the same time collecting their outrageous underfunded pensions. Remember the fate of Mr. Mulroney. He won his first election by admonishing Mr. Turner about Mr. Trudeau's patronage. Unfortunately Mr. Mulroney's patronage largesse outdid that of his predecessors and in my opinion contributed to the electoral disaster of the Conservative party.

Lobbyists:

These individuals represent special interests and attempt to sway politicians to support these interests. Their clients' interest may not be in the best interest of the country as a whole. Many lobbyists are well connected politically and for this reason are engaged by their clients. Apparently some of their fees are on a contingency basis. Why is it permissible for lobbyists but illegal for lawyers to obtain a large piece of the action when their efforts are successful? I have never seen figures on the cost of lobbying to the taxpayer but suspect that it is substantial. During the campaign your party stated that supplicants to the government did not need lobbyists to get a fair hearing. Mr. Chrétien has stated repeatedly that lobbyists are going to be more accountable. So far little has been done.

Senate:

This subject could be considered under the paragraph on patronage since essentially all Senate appointment are made by this method. *Most Canadians would agree that the Senate is a costly irrelevant body and should be changed or abolished. MacLeans October 10 issue had an excellent article by Diane Francis with a worthy idea by Frank Stronach. He proposes replacing senators with "Citizens Representatives." Enclosed is a copy of the Article for your information. I like the idea so much that if I were elected as a citizens representative I would serve without pay. If I were asked to become a senator, I would decline the opportunity.*

If these areas—i.e., exorbitant pensions, patronage appointments, lobbyists, and senate—were corrected, many millions of dollars would be saved and in addition you would demonstrate your leadership ability to the country.

Alberta's Premier Ralph Klein has applied major cuts to many areas of expense. In doing so his popularity with his electorate has increased. I suggest that you review his expense reductions and borrow many of his ideas.

Social Programs:

You as well as Mr. Axworthy have stated that social programs must be changed. Unemployment insurance is not fair to many stable industries and is abused by other industries such as fishing. Foreign Aid should be reviewed—why for example should we have recently given $30 million of borrowed money to Haiti?

Over-government:

As Canadians we are substantially over-governed at the federal, provincial and municipal levels. Duplication of services necessitates excess government employees with, like politicians, overgenerous pensions. Substantial savings should result from elimination of duplication. I can't see for example why you cannot over-ride the reluctance of the provinces to integrate the PST and GST.

Regional Development Agencies and Farm Marketing Boards:

All of these should be reviewed to determine whose best interest they represent. I am cynical enough to suspect that they are in the best interest of the mandarins who administer them as well as perhaps in some cases the farm producers. Most certainly they are not in the best interests of the consumer and the taxpayer.

Business Subsidies:

In many cases these subsidies have been a disaster to the taxpayer. Petro Canada is a good example. This ill conceived state owned company (now 70 percent) has written off over 2 billion dollars of taxpayers' money as a bad investment.

Massey Ferguson had a gigantic government bailout and was subsequently downsized and renamed Varity. After the company received this government largesse, it moved to Buffalo. According to its president, Victor Rice, the main reasons for leaving Canada were high taxes and government left-wing policies. In the past four years since leaving Canada, the company has increased its market capitalization from 100 million to 2 billion. It seems to me that the contract with Massey Ferguson should have included a clause requiring repayment of the loan if the company decided to leave Canada.

Recently Royal Oak Mines made the decision to move from Vancouver to Seattle. Other Canadian companies are considering moving to the USA or offshore because of high taxes and government over-regulation. We simply cannot afford to drive industry out of Canada. To keep jobs in Canada we need the lowest possible tax rate and the highest possible tax base. We do not need large infusion of tax dollars into moribund industries.

Streamline Government Departments:

All government departments should be carefully scrutinized for excess spending. I have no doubt that substantial reductions in the numbers of civil servants could be made without affecting the business of the country. In order to remain competitive many industries have had to downsize their staff. Surely governments could duplicate this strategy.

Privatization of Prisons:

Several American states have contracted out operation of prisons to the private sector. It is my understanding that prisons operated by the private sector function at a cost substantially below that of government institutions. An investigation should be undertaken to ascertain whether or not such a system would benefit Canada.

Amusement subsidized by Governments:

It is my opinion that if Canadians want to be entertained it should be paid for by themselves rather than by various levels of government.

Let us consider the following:

(1) By allowing many sports event tickets, such as to baseball games, hockey games, etc. to be eligible as tax deductions, we in effect subsidize overpaid athletes. Let these sports stand on their own merit or fold because without government tax subsidy ticket costs would rise. If the Ontario government had not wasted 350 million dollars it is unlikely the Sky Dome would have been built.

(2) Amateur sports needs to be reassessed. Do we need such edifices as the Ottawa multi-million "Disneyland of Blair Road" for the administration of amateur sports? I am not convinced that we should fund amateur sports when money is desperately needed in other areas.

(3) The same reasoning should apply to other areas of amusement, such as theatre, ballet, symphony, etc. If patrons of such functions want to retain their pleasure, they should be prepared to pay whatever it costs in their ticket price (now deductible). Remember that most taxpayers now subsidizing all the above amusements do not attend in person.

Health Care:

Sooner or later the health care issue will have to be addressed, since it is not affordable in its present form. Most past and present politicians for vote getting purposes regard this issue as a "sacred cow" and therefore untouchable. Substantial savings would be realized by imposing a modest user fee on those who could afford such users fee. Consider what premiums car insurance companies would have to charge if there were no deductible. Every minor scratch would have to be repaired at no charge to the user. Another possible change would be to add back as taxable income all or part of the annual medical cost incurred by users of the health care system.

The Quebec Issue:

I hope that if and when the Quebec referendum takes place the people of Quebec vote to stay in Canada. I do not believe that the rest of Canada should bribe the people of Quebec to stay. Rather they should want to stay as equal partners with the rest of the provinces. They should be allowed to retain their individuality with respect to language, laws, etc. Since Confederation, multi-billion dollars have been thrown at Quebec to keep the voters happy. This largesse should not be exacerbated.

I further believe that bilingualism has been a financial disaster for Canada. Bilingualism should not be countrywide, but rather the second official language should be available to communities where numbers warrant such expense.

Immigration:

Recently I wrote a letter to Mr. Rock and Mr. Marchi, a copy of which is enclosed, making suggestions in gun control and immigration changes. I am pleased that Mr. Marchi's statement on November 1 included a number of my suggestions. It is my opinion that if and when enacted into law Mr. Marchi's changes will result in substantial savings that will assist you in reducing the deficit.

Ottawa Cheque writers must work overtime:

Enclosed for your information is an article by William Watson which was published in the October 28 Financial Post. *Mr. Martin, I hope that your axe is very sharp when you decimate these onerous expenditures. When I see the amounts spent on such ridiculous grants, I am convinced that your good business sense should guide you.*

I wish you well in your most difficult task. No doubt you will be inundated with advice on how to cut the deficit. No doubt most advisors will want spending cuts in areas not affecting themselves. Be severe, and be fair. Don't forget to be a leader, as suggested in my opening remarks. I hope that my suggestions (I could make many more) will be of some use in your deliberations.

To the Honourable Paul Martin

Yours very truly,
J.E.B. Graham D.V.M.

copies to:
Axworthy, Lloyd, Minister of Human Resources
Bouchard, Lucien, Leader of Opposition
Chrétien, Jean P., Prime Minister of Canada
Corcoran, Terence, The Globe and Mail
Doering, Charles CFRB Toronto
Francis, Diane, Editor, Financial Post
Manning, Preston, Leader Reform Party Canada
Harris, Mike, Leader, Ontario Progressive Conservative
Party
Marchi, Sergio Immigration Minister
Peters, Douglas, M.P. Scarborough East
Rae, Bob, Premier Ontario
Rock, Allan, Minister of Justice
Somerville, David, National Citizens Coalition
Watson, William, Financial Post
Others, Friends and acquaintances whom I will encourage to support my view

The text of Mr. Martin's response is offered:

December 2, 1994
   Thank you for your recent representation concerning our financial situation and what the government should do to improve it. Your comments and suggestions have been noted. Canadians continue to express concern about our nation's finances and this is certainly understandable. Although the deficit is still higher than it should be, stronger economic growth is having a positive effect.
   Nonetheless, we must continue to find ways to improve our situation even more. That is why represen-

tations like yours are important: they help us to identify the issues that concern Canadians most and to focus our efforts toward solutions. As I trust you will appreciate, we simply cannot do or be all things. Therefore, having to make choices is unavoidable. Of course, we want to make the right decisions so your input is useful in help-ing us to determine the direction we must take.

I am pleased to have had this opportunity to correspond with you.

> *Sincerely,*
> *The Honourable Paul Martin, P.C., M.P.*

Mr. Martin mentioned that representations such as mine are important. If, however, one considers the various points that I raised as well as the subsequent events, little has been done to stem the flow of the money derived from Canadian tax-payers and wasted in the ways that I suggested. Currently as prime minister he is trying to overcome the fallout from the misuse of taxpayers' funds in the province of Quebec. If he had, as finance minister, implemented some of my suggestions, this malfeasance could have been prevented. If he is still prime minister after the election expected soon, perhaps he should again read my correspondence.

Subsequent to his letter Mr. Martin is credited with reduc-ing the deficit to zero. Many financial experts are of the opinion that this change was mainly due to the federal government off-loading expenses to the provinces and to the municipalities. In addition, the trade balance with the USA due to the Free Trade Agreement can be credited with part of the deficit reduction.

Chapter Thirty-Five

My Worst Nightmare

A nightmare can express a feeling of impending doom.

Over the years I have had many nightmares, often associated with being pursued by tigers, lions, grizzly bears, and so on. One night in October 2003, I had the most frightening nightmare of all. In my dream I was the soon to be ex-prime minister of Canada, ousted by my own party and my long-time nemesis, Paul Martin. What a way to end my career! I decided that I would continue to feather my own nest as has been my custom. Here is my thought-process:

> *Since it is inevitable that Paul Martin will soon be prime minister, I must think of a suitable legacy so that the people of Canada will remember me. I will start with what should be done for my current cabinet ministers, as well as others of my entourage, who have been helpful to me during my years in office. It is unlikely that many of my current cabinet ministers will be invited to become*

ministers in Martin's cabinet. This means that I will have to reward them for their loyalty to me. It will tax even my ingenuity to provide comfy positions for all of them. More important than my loyalty to them, I have to provide a suitable position for myself.

By never admitting a mistake I have had wonderful success during my political career. My first priority will be to provide immunity for myself in the event that the RCMP gathers enough evidence to charge me with malfeasance.

My second priority will be to use my talents to supplement my generous pension to be provided by future taxpayers. I am aware that unlike ordinary taxpayers, many of whom have to save for their own retirement, the pensions of retired politicians are essentially unfunded.

In order to accomplish this I have decided, while I still control my cabinet, to set up a new consulting position for myself. I will call it "The Ethics Czar," or some such name. It will report only to me, as does Mr. Wilson at present. Unilaterally I can stonewall any criticism. My current cabinet will go along with my ideas, since without me they will receive no favours. With all my experience in hiding questionable situations, I believe that I have the talents for such a position. As a matter of fact, I believe that I am unique in Canada with so much experience. I am sure that I could teach such a university course to Ph.D. aspirants.

My clients could come from all walks of life, including politicians, biker gang members, crooked company executives, etcetera. It would be imperative for me to have the power to personally grant tax certificates to my clients who will take advantage of my expensive consulting fees. Speaking of taxes, my own pension as well as my expected very lucrative consulting business will be excluded from paying the onerous income taxes that I have imposed on Canadians. I am sure that this exemption can be arranged, as was the case for certain rich families from Quebec. Obviously all of this, particularly tax exemptions, will have to be arranged prior to Martin becoming prime minister. As an ex-finance minister, he would be unlikely to provide such a benefit for me.

The Canadian Government must supply suitable office accommodation for me. My preferred location would be on the Hull side of the Ottawa River. This would necessitate a tunnel under the river in order that the Martin cabinet ministers could consult me without being caught. My office would be luxurious, in keeping with my status. I envision the roof as the location for my putting green and driving range. This area would of course have a retractable roof, similar to the one on the Sky Dome. All of this seems to be expensive, however if you consider how I blew one hundred million dollars to purchase two Bombardier jet airplanes for my personal use as well as for the use of cabinet ministers, and said to be unnecessary by my defence department, it would be cheap. Also my government wasted a billion or more on gun control (the original estimate was a couple of million; I don't know what happened to escalate the cost) but in retrospect it was doomed from the start. When these and all the other examples of government waste are considered, the cost of my new digs could not be considered unreasonable.

I will discuss these as well as other nefarious matters with my golfing buddy, Bill Clinton. I admire the way he pardoned about 140 people of various offences, just before he left office. How about Marc Rich, who was convicted in 1983 of defrauding the IRS of forty-eight million dollars? Rather than face trial, he fled to Switzerland and allowed his wife in the USA to continue contributing to Bill's campaigns in the amount of several hundred thousand dollars. Bill pardoned his half-brother of various charges including narcotics violations and influence peddling. I admire Bill for his gall and for the fact that he got away with it. There was also his affair with Monica that I can't agree with in case Aline reads these musings.

I must phone Bill, since he is an expert in some of the matters my consultant's job will involve. Maybe he will do this for me as a favour rather than bill me at his ridiculous fee schedule. As a matter of fact, he and I, working together, could put on a series of seminars related to our expertise.

Sometimes I wonder if I should consult a psychiatrist. One of the Canadian bishops said recently that I may end up in Hell because of my stand on homosexuality. Also the Vatican would not go along with my wish to send one of my fallen ex-cabinet ministers to Rome. In addition, many people will not like the idea of my future career. I do have some regret that waste by my government cut down on the funds needed for health care.

I doubt that Paul Martin would approve of the expenditures related to my retirement. His followers should know by now that I cannot leave office until my new business is organized.

It would be fair to say that this nightmare was more frightening than being chased by large carnivores. In that case I would be the only victim! In this scenario, the Canadian taxpayers would continue to be excessively penalized by the Little Guy from Quebec.

Chapter Thirty-Six

Political Crisis: The Canadian Taxpayers Have Been Milked Again

Since some of my readers may not be familiar with the secessionist movement, the following is a brief description of the principals of the Quebec referendum of 1995.

The secessionist movement in Quebec felt that it had enough support to win a province-wide referendum and with a majority vote could legally negotiate with Canada to secede and form a separate country. A "Yes" vote would have given Quebec governments a powerful club that could be used as a threat in any negotiations with Canada. The referendum received the support of 49.4 percent of the vote. Approximately 53,499 more votes (in about six million) in favour of separation may have resulted in the dissolution of the country, and Canada would have suffered a substantial loss.

Presumably as a method to avoid another referendum, the then prime minister, Jean Chrétien, decided to appease poten-tial secessionists by bribing the province of Quebec with largesse from general funds, i.e., taxpayer dollars from the rest of Canada. Included in this gesture was much questionable benevolence. Alphonso Gagliano, a cabinet minister, was Quebec Lieutenant responsible for carrying out the prime minister's orders. Gagliano was an accountant by profession and was alleged to have members of the Mafia as clients. It seems that this should have been considered prior to his appointment. He was in charge of hiring several advertising agencies who received huge commissions, often for little or no work. A large part of these commissions were donated back to the Liberal Party. These fraudulent activities went on for several years.

Sheila Fraser, Auditor General for Canada, in late 2003 revealed some of these nefarious activities. On February 10, 2004, her major report was released to Parliament and to the press. The report understandably resulted in consternation throughout Canada.

Her disclosure has demonstrated many areas of negligent behavior, as well as outright fraud, that encompassed not only individuals and private companies but also some Crown corporations, such as the post office, Via Rail, and even the Administrative Branch of the RCMP. The Business Development Bank, another Crown corporation, was approached by the then prime minister, Chrétien, to advance financing for a hotel that was adjacent to a golf course in which he had a financial interest. This golf course depended on golfers from this hotel for income. In spite of reluctance to provide the loan, the president of the bank was forced to comply. When the loan became questionable, he wanted to foreclose and was overruled by political pressure. The bank president was fired from his position and was alleged to have been dishonest in the management of bank funds. He sued for wrongful dismissal and was successful. The judge hearing the case wrote that the bank was pressured and that the man's reputation was severely damaged. The cost of this litigation offers another example of government waste. This case has been under investigation by the RCMP for several years.

The new prime minister, Paul Martin, immediately called for a judicial inquiry that will be asked to determine the extent of the malfeasance. Many will be required to testify. We all hope that the inquiry will determine the extent of the problem and that remedies can be put in place to prevent a recurrence of the most scandalous event in the history of Canada. I decided to write the following e-mail to Paul Martin, our new prime minister, to express my concerns. My letter, in part, appears below:

February 17, 2004

The Right Honourable Paul Martin
Prime Minister of Canada

Dear Sir:
During the past thirty years I have written many letters to politicians, mostly related to waste of taxpayers' money. Some of these letters, including one to you dated November 7, 1994, as well as your reply of December 2, 1994, are included in the revision of my autobiography, entitled Sow's Ear To Silk Purse—Anecdotes from the Life of a Veterinarian. *This edition is scheduled for publication in the summer of 2004. Soon after you became minister of finance you requested input from Canadians for ideas on how to reduce the deficit. I made several suggestions, such as withdrawing the "gold plated" pension benefit for politicians, making lobbyists more accountable, eliminating patronage appointments, withdrawing tax benefits for tickets to sporting events, and several other suggestions. In addition I sent you copies of a letter I wrote to Mr. Rock and Mr. Marchi on the combined subjects of immigration and gun control. Both of these issues now cost the taxpayers large amounts of money. I suggested in my letter that gun control was bad legislation in that it penalized sportsmen, farmers, and sustenance*

hunters rather than criminals who use illegal weapons and who would be unlikely to register such weapons. Who would have thought that rather than the initial estimate of two million dollars the cost would escalate to more than a billion! Could it be more inept management?

Sheila Fraser, the auditor general, has amazed and shocked Canadians with her discovery of incompetence and fraudulent activities by some members of the Liberal Party. One such master of unacceptable behavior is Mr. Gagliano, whom you relieved last week of his duties in Denmark. You stated that he will not receive severance pay. It is probable that he will need no such payment. It is ironic that Mr. Chrétien wanted him to have the plum post of Ambassador to the Vatican. The Vatican is to be congratulated for refusing this overture.

You have announced that there will be a judicial inquiry to delve into the allegations of incompetence and fraud. Presumably those giving testimony under oath will include Mr. Gagliano and Mr. Chrétien, as well as numerous underlings, perhaps even more than the few you have suggested. It is my opinion that the inquiry should include all of those, including Mr. Gagliano's staff, whose testimony would be important. It would be most helpful to the inquiry if you were to grandfather the whistle-blower act that you have promised to enact. Individuals would be less reluctant to testify when they enjoy protection. It would also demonstrate that you are abandoning the dictatorial philosophy of your predecessor. You have stated that those who are guilty will be punished. You have also stated that there is something rotten in the Liberal Party. You, as prime minister, must correct these problems or be prepared to endure the wrath of the voters.

The integrity of the Canadian political system must be restored. Blatant disregard of the taxpayers' hard-earned money must be rectified. Those who abused the system must be punished with appropriate penalties as well as the refunding of the spoils of their criminal activity. Should any cabinet minister, or a prime minister be found guilty, the title Honourable or Right Honourable should be permanently revoked. If these titles are left with convicted parties, the title will lose all respect of the citizens.

The RCMP as well as other Crown Corporations was included as being part of this massive fraud. Apparently the administrative branch, but not the criminal branch, was involved and the criminal branch should be able to continue their investigation of the Shawinigate and other matters. Perhaps it will be easier for them now that there is a new Prime Minister.

I find it difficult to accept that you, as finance minister as well as vice president of the treasury board, could have been unaware of the malfeasance rampant in Quebec. As finance minister you collect the money, and as vice president you should have ensured that it was properly spent...

It is my considered opinion that you should avoid calling an election prior to the release of the findings of the judicial inquiry in order to satisfy the voters that you, unlike other Liberals, played no part in this debacle. A premature election call would be unacceptable.

Sincerely,
   J.E.B. Graham DVM

Copies of this e-mail will be sent to the following:
Editor, The Globe and Mail
Editor, the National Post
Editor, the Ottawa Citizen
Dr. Grant Hill, Interim Leader, the Conservative Party
Dr. Carolyn Bennett MP
Jack Layton, leader, NDP Party

It seems doubtful that Mr. Martin ever saw my letter. For answer I received a standard form reply, included below:

Dear J.E.B. Graham:

On behalf of the Right Honourable Paul Martin, I wish to acknowledge receipt of your e-mail.

The time you have taken to write on the recent report from the Auditor General (AG) is appreciated. The Prime Minister was deeply troubled by the findings of the AG. Indeed, this report paints a disturbing picture that, simply put, the Government finds unacceptable.

As such, one of the first actions of the new Government was to abolish the sponsorship program. Furthermore, as soon as the report was made available, the Government acted promptly with a series of measures to address all of the AG's concerns and recommendations, as follows:

—The creation of an Independent Commission of Public Inquiry to investigate and examine all remaining questions relating to the sponsorship and advertising programs;

—Steps to ensure that the House of Commons Public Accounts Committee chaired by an Opposition Member is being struck early so that it can begin the important work of receiving and reviewing the Auditor General's report;

—The appointment of Mr. André Gauthier as Special Counsel for financial recovery with a mandate to pursue all possible avenues, including civil litigation, to recover funds improperly received by certain parties;

—The enacting of reforms of government departments and Crown corporations based on gaps highlighted in the report, so that we can ensure it never happens again.

The auditor general has acknowledged that a number of corrective actions have been taken already by the government, but it is determined to do much more. We will ensure that ethical standards and management practices in the federal public sector are raised even higher.

Accordingly, the government will introduce legislation to protect whistleblowers, mandate changes to the governance of Crown corporations that fall under the Financial Administration Act (FAA), report on proposed changes to the FAA and on the respective responsibilities and accountabilities of Ministers and public servants as recommended by the AG.

You may be assured that the concerns you have raised have been carefully noted. The Prime Minister always appreciates hearing from Canadians.

Thank you for writing to the Prime Minister.

L.A. Lavell
Executive Correspondence Officer
Agent de correspondence de la haute direction

As it happens, I had also written a letter on December 1, 2003, to Dr. Carolyn Bennett, a colleague of Mr. Martin, and Member for our riding, requesting advice regarding tax rebates in connection with the publication of this book. At publication date I had not received from her even a standard form reply. One is tempted to wonder how often politicians read their mail.

Big Trout
Conservation Club

Chapter Thirty-Seven

Big Trout Conservation Club

In early May, 1959, I was invited to be a guest at a private fishing lodge located in central Ontario halfway between Orillia and Minden. The lodge had been in operation for many years, catering to guests for fishing and deer hunting.

We left our cars and climbed on an old army truck for the six-mile trip to Long Lake. A bush road built as a maintenance road for a power line was the only land access to the site. This road, undoubtedly the worst road I have ever travelled, required a four-wheel drive vehicle to crawl over the rocks and through various beaver ponds. We transferred our equipment to wooden boats for the remainder of the trip to the fishing camp.

Located at the junction of Long Lake and Big Trout Lake, the camp consisted of a frame building used as a kitchen, living area, and sleeping accommodation. The beds, upper and lower bunks at one end of the building, accommodated twelve men. The facilities were somewhat less than ostentatious, the privy, strictly an outdoor model!

Our group had five guests as well as the owner, Roy Windover. Soon after arrival we split up two to a boat and began to fish for lake trout. The boats were homemade wooden craft and seemed to be seaworthy. In the early spring, lake trout are usually found near the surface. As the water gets warmer the trout move to deeper water, since they need a water temperature of 40 to 45 degrees Fahrenheit for survival. While this was the first time I had fished for lake trout, anything that I had read about this species intimated that they were very hard to catch. Before long we all started to catch trout and soon had our daily limit.

After our evening meal, one of our group decided that he would crawl into his upper bunk. He had imbibed too much and accidentally bumped into a nail projecting from the ceiling, suffering a large wound that extended around one eye from top to bottom. Luckily, only the skin was involved. We decided that the wound repair should be done in the camp. Since there was no medical doctor with us, a dentist and I volunteered. First we increased the level of alcohol in his system and then applied ice packs to the wound. Next we sterilized a darning needle and some nylon fishing line to use as suture material. The alcohol and ice pack worked very well as anaesthetic, and the repair was accomplished. We advised him to see his physician as soon as possible after our return to civilization. His doctor felt that the procedure looked fine and nothing more needed to be done. I saw the chap a year later and noticed only the faintest trace of a scar. Over the years we improved our first aid kit with proper surgical instruments, suture material, and better analgesics.

The following year, I, as well as a number of other new recruits, was invited on another fishing trip to the camp. It became an annual outing. Some of us decided to try deer hunting—an annual November event. Deer were very numerous in the area. The best part of this activity, from my point of view, was the fellowship. The group included physicians, a lawyer, real-estate people, and three veterinarians, as well as invitees from various other walks of life.

A group of eight men including myself decided to buy the camp from Roy Windover and change it from the previous semi-commercial operation to a private club. Roy's father had started to come to Big Trout Lake many years before and had owned a site on the lake a short distance from our camp. He had sold this property and had leased the land for the current camp from the provincial government. The lease was for a hunting camp and was renewed on an annual basis. This presented a problem, since there was no guarantee of long-term security.

A friend of mine, Ken Giles, was a salesman for an X-ray company, and our veterinary practice was in his territory. Ken and I had similar farming backgrounds. Both of us enjoyed the outdoors. He and I carried out the original negotiations with Roy and were instrumental in Big Trout becoming a members' club. The men in the initial core group were all close friends and all felt that we could work together in harmony. Eventually the group increased to twelve members, with each new member coming in on the recommendation of one of the existing members.

Gordon Teskey, a lawyer and one of the first members, drew up the original constitution. One of the provisions was that any potential new member must have unanimous acceptance. One dissenting vote precluded admission. As a close-knit group we wanted to avoid contention.

The deer-hunting season always started on the first Monday in November. The men usually arrived a day or two early so that the necessary work such as getting supplies to camp, cutting firewood, etc., could be accomplished. We developed a tradition. On the evening prior to the hunt, we conducted a meeting that always included lectures on safety. One presentation was on safety in the camp, underlining the provision that no loaded gun could be brought into the building. There had been an incident in which a guest who was not a member was cleaning his rifle in the camp when it discharged. Fortunately no one was injured. This guest was immediately asked to leave and was never invited to return. Care with respect to boats was raised, since this method of transportation was used in almost all of the trips from the camp to hunting areas. Many hunters have drowned because of overloaded boats.

The third safety issue included responsibility of the hunters in the bush. Each had to know exactly where the man on either side was stationed. In addition, a deer had to be precisely identified before a shot could be fired. Taking alcohol into the bush was prohibited. While all of us had listened to these rules on many occasions, repetition was welcomed. During the many years that I hunted with this group, we never had a serious accident.

Late in the afternoon, after the day's hunt, any deer that had been harvested were brought back to the camp. The animals were field dressed in the bush and returned in the boats. One of the veterinarians, usually me, had the job of washing the carcasses with a hose fed by a pump in the lake. A careful inspection would be made to assure that no gross evidence of any disease process was present. Any imperfections in the field dressing were corrected, and the deer would be hung on a pole with the rear end near the ground to allow drainage. Handled in this manner, the meat was always well preserved.

Card games such as euchre, bridge, or poker occupied our evenings. Since the day would start at 5:00 a.m., most of the hunters retired early. We usually had a cook to prepare the meals and most times had an assistant to the cook, responsible for washing the dishes, peeling the vegetables, and keeping the camp tidy.

During the mid 1960s, our group decided to expand the camp. We constructed a new building for sleeping accommodation with beds for sixteen men. It had a bathroom with two sinks and a shower stall. Outdoor privies were built for normal use, and an indoor toilet that was supposed to be used as a night emergency facility. This additional building was long overdue and made camp life much more comfortable. The original building was adapted for enlarged living room space as well as more room in the dining area. A fireplace was installed to give supplementary heat to that provided by the wood stove heaters. The kitchen was modernized with a propane cook stove and propane refrigerators. Bringing in all of the building materials as well as refrigerators, stoves, and other equipment presented a monumental task. We purchased aluminum boats to replace the old wooden boats. Another small building provided sleeping accommodations for a further five men.

From time to time, poaching of fish and deer became a problem. The remoteness of the camp rendered inspection by game wardens infrequent. An old farm with 100 acres of property was offered for sale. This farm was the last deeded property before crown land that extended all the way to our camp. In addition, the power line right of way mentioned earlier passed through the centre of the farm. Working together, five of us purchased the property. As soon as we got possession we constructed a massive steel gate at the entrance to our property with signs saying "Private Property—No Admittance." We felt that we could help the game wardens reduce the poaching activity. Before long, local citizens started a massive letter-writing campaign, the letters being sent to representatives for the federal and provincial ridings. We were told that there had never been such a protest over any issue in that area. Various people approached us, requesting that we remove the barrier. We declined. Eventually we offered the provincial representatives a deal: we would deed them the right of way in exchange for title to the property occupied by our camp. They declined this offer, since the one negotiating with us did not have the power to make the deal. A few weeks later the same man came to my home, since I was the negotiator, and suggested that the government might cancel the lease on our camp and turn the property into a bird sanctuary. Annoyed by this threat, I took his name and told him that his comment would be related to his superiors.

In the meantime, the ministry had received bids on the cost of constructing a road around our property to satisfy the local opposition. The new road required a bridge over a large creek; the cost was estimated at $400,000.00. This was too costly for consideration by the government, so our negotiations resumed. One of the members of our camp had a friend, a lawyer influential with the existing provincial government. An appointment was made for me to meet with this gentleman. I prepared a brief that demonstrated some of the things our group had done to help the ministry and the environment and discussed with him the threat made by the provincial representative. He told me that he would see what could be done. In a little more than a week I was invited to the Minden office of the Ministry of Natural Resources to review the problem. They offered to make the land exchange (at their cost), provided that we would allow them to maintain an existing portage between Long Lake and Big Trout Lake. This portage would be on our new property. We felt that this was a small price to pay and were satisfied. We had tried for many years to get title to the property, and finally it had happened.

During the early years of our Big Trout Association, snowmobiles were becoming popular. Early one February six of our members decided to try this new winter activity and decided to spend a weekend at our camp fishing for lake trout. This decision necessitated reserving rental machines as well as towed sleds to transport necessities from Minden to Big Trout Lake, a distance of about seven miles. None of us had any experience with these machines, but we were all willing to try our luck.

We all, with one exception, purchased appropriate cold-weather clothing for this adventure. The one exception decided to use his deer hunting garments. While suitable for November weather, this apparel was not adequate for February temperatures.

Late on a Friday afternoon we made the two-hour drive from Toronto to Minden. We signed up for our rental machines and sleds and started on our trip. We soon found that the bush with snow on the ground looks very different from what it is in November. Just before darkness set in, we missed the turn off the main trail to go to our lake. We made the decision to return to Minden to ask one of our members to act as our guide and to assist us in navigation. This man was enjoying the comfort of his home on this bitterly cold night but agreed to help. We started on the second trip and noted as we left that the temperature was now forty degrees below zero Fahrenheit.

We were all young and strong so in spite of the temperature decided to try again. When we finally reached Long Lake, which we had to cross to get to Big Trout Lake, we opted to have a rest stop and enjoy a beer. Opening the case of beer, we were greatly dismayed to find that all of the bottles had frozen and split. Being resourceful, we turned to our whisky bottle. By now it was very dark, and the chap pouring the liquor said there was some obstruction preventing the flow. Someone produced a flashlight and we found that while this bottle was not broken, it was full of ice crystals that prevented the flow. So much for good liquor!

It was a short trip, about fifteen minutes, to the camp, where we could start a fire to warm up the booze as well as our precooked supper. The inside of our camp was, like the outside, forty below. We were able to light the propane stove to warm up the supper as well as light the stove to warm up the building. While the stove seemed, at the time, to make the camp more comfortable, during the two days we were there the highest temperature we attained was about thirty degrees Fahrenheit. The snow from our boots on the floor never melted.

The primary purpose of this expedition was lake trout fishing. To accomplish this we had to cut holes through three feet of ice. For all of this preparation, hardship, and time spent fishing, we caught not a single lake trout!

I mentioned that one of our members had inadequate cold weather protection. Soon after we got back to Toronto, he was hospitalized with pneumonia. Happily he made a good recovery.

Would I ever undertake such an excursion again? It has been said that experience is a great teacher. I believe I got the point of this lesson!

When Janet was old enough to look after herself, Barbara and I often went to Big Trout Lake. Prior to that she would accompany us and bring Mandy, our little French poodle, for company. One hot summer afternoon, Barbara, Mandy, and I arrived at the camp after an exhausting trip over the bad road. Dirt in the gas line had caused frequent stalling. Usually when we arrived we would unload the equipment and do a little lake trout fishing. Since we intended to stay for a week, we decided to take it easy for the evening. Since the camp had not been used for some time, some chores had to be done, including lighting the propane refrigerator, the cook stove, and the hot water heaters in the kitchen and sleeping cabin. I proceeded to look after these jobs, and Barbara sat down at the piano and provided some music.

An explosion from the direction of the sleeping cabin startled us. I went to investigate. It took only a few seconds to reach the building. I opened the door of the cabin.

Fire!

The hot water tank had exploded; flames were already shooting to the ceiling. I ran outside and shut off the propane tank. The propane-fed fire had spread to the rafters in the ceiling. By this time Barbara had arrived to help with the problem. The water supply to the buildings is pumped from the lake to an elevated holding tank, and the water then runs by gravity to the faucets. With a short ladder I was able to access the flames in the ceiling while Barbara filled buckets of water from the sinks and from the shower. We soon got the flames out.

Since considerable charring of the wood had occurred, we watched for further eruption of the flames; fortunately none occurred. One of our camp rules required that the water tank be filled prior to leaving. Had this not been the case, it is likely that all of the camp buildings would have been lost. We went to Minden the next day to report the fire to the insurance agency, then returned to the camp. The thermostat to the propane water heater was found to be defective and had not shut off when the water reached the proper temperature.

During the deer hunting weeks, numerous practical jokes were played. My room, which I shared with three others, had a decrepit bearskin. We decided to discard it and took it to our dump, situated on a hill above and behind the camp. We hung the skin over a sawhorse. Even in daylight looked quite realistic. We targeted one very gullible friend for the prank. This chap had always wanted to shoot a bear, but the opportunity to do so had never arisen. If we could persuade him that there was a bear on the dump, he would jump at the chance. He had been the target of many pranks, so he was rather suspicious.

The cook's assistant was asked to announce, after the evening meal was finished and the men were relaxing in the sleeping area, that he had taken the food scraps to the dump and had seen a large bear feeding on the waste. All of the hunters except the victim were aware that the prank was to occur. I asked if anyone would like to shoot the bear, since we did not want the animal so close to our quarters. Bob immediately jumped up and offered to get rid of our problem bear. I said, "Well, to prevent an accident only one man may bring a rifle, and anyone who wishes to come must stay behind Bob. I will carry the flashlight and lead the group up the hill."

Upon arrival at the dump, I moved the light back and forth. When the light shone on the skin, I moved it. After several passes Bob shouted, "There it is—hold the light still or you will get us all killed." I obliged and held the light on the target. After the loud bang, I pushed the muzzle of the gun toward the sky. One of our buddies picked up the skin and commented: "Bob that was a hell of a shot; you skinned him!" Poor Bob—again a victim!

Clients, friends, and acquaintances often asked me, "Why would you, a veterinarian, go deer hunting?" The normal answer was, "I enjoy eating properly prepared game and am of the opinion that there is little difference between eating venison and beef." The argument that beef evolves from a domesticated animal rather than a wild animal is not valid in my opinion. I enjoyed my deer hunting trips mainly for the social interaction with good friends. The friends made through this group are still included as my best friends.

It should be realized that life could have been lost if the hunters had disobeyed the safety laws mentioned earlier. During a time of need, each member would do whatever was necessary to help his friend. On several occasions someone needed assistance, including financial assistance, and this was given without question. Last but not least, the camp was a getaway place from the stress of a busy practice. After a few days in the bush, I always returned rejuvenated.

During the early 1960s the deer population peaked. At that time it was permissible to take any deer, be it buck, doe, or fawn. As a personal preference, I permitted the does and fawns to tread quietly past my watch. In time the deer population began to dwindle. Several reasons accounted for this. Deer require the branches of young trees for a substantial part of their food; as the bush matured it was harder for them to reach their food supply. Several predators, including timber wolves and black bears, played a part in reducing the population. One interesting study was done on black bears taken during the spring hunting season. Post-mortems of these bears showed that about 40 percent had either fawns or juvenile moose in their stomachs. To a lesser degree, the hunters probably played a role, although the argument was made that prior to 1960 there were just as many hunters during deer season and the deer were plentiful. Competition from moose should be considered a factor. Moose will graze on bushes as well as marsh grasses. When they feed on trees, since they are larger than deer they can reach higher. By so doing they compete with the deer for food. In my first years of deer hunting, it was very unusual to see a moose. Now they are numerous in the area.

I often think about the early years of our group at Big Trout Lake. Many of the original members, as well as some who joined later, are no longer with us. Ed Teachman, an engineer from Hamilton, was one of the founders. While his marksmanship ability was doubtful, he was a great buddy. He is remembered for donating an upright piano to the camp. The transportation of this instrument over terrible roads as well as its ride in a boat is a club legend. One of our guys, Bob Taylor, also now deceased, played the piano on that boat trip. The animals in the bush must have pricked up their ears when they heard the strange sounds. Bob is also remembered as the recipient of practical jokes, including shooting the bear skin.

Dr. Barry Woods, a radiologist from Oshawa, also now departed, has been replaced as a member by his son, Dr. Donald Woods, a family physician. One evening during the early years of our group, Barry visited our home. He was returning from Windsor where he had purchased an airplane on floats. He was very excited about this new hobby and had arranged to take his first flying lesson the following weekend. On Monday morning I read in the newspaper a story about a float plane that had crashed in a lake while attempting to land. It was Barry, and he had severe fractures to both ankles. The repair was only partly successful, and he had to use canes most of his remaining days. When Barry purchased the plane, he was told that the insurance was transferable. He had one trip in the plane and found out after the fact that the insurance was not transferable. As well as his injuries he suffered a substantial financial loss. In spite of his handicap, he maintained his interest in fishing.

Doctor Luke Teskey, a general surgeon and brother of Gordon Teskey our resident lawyer, was a great addition to the camp. He always brought his black bag full of equipment to be used in case of emergency. Luke developed viral hepatitis, contracted from a patient during an operation. He did not respond to treatment. He had a liver transplant and passed away approximately one year later. His brother, Gordon, is now a tax court judge for Canada and travels extensively to fulfill this position. It is always a pleasure to see Gord for golf, bridge, or a fishing trip.

Two of my good friends, both veterinarians, Dr Len Burch and Dr. Holt Webster, have also passed away. In addition to being a good veterinarian, Len was very skilled as a carpenter. When he moved from Scarborough to Minden, he built his own house. Len was musically minded as well, played the guitar and knew the words of many country music songs. He died at a young age as the result of a heart attack.

Holt was a jolly fellow and well liked. Our veterinary group bought his animal hospital when he retired from active practice. Holt was an ardent fisherman and spent many days at Big Trout. He and his wife Phyllys purchased a mobile home and like gypsies travelled the continent. Holt died of a brain tumour. He and I shared many delightful days.

Gordon Hanna was a general contractor. His skills were a useful addition to our group for the maintenance of our buildings. He developed severe sneezing spells, diagnosed as a sinus infection. When he failed to respond to treatment, his nasal passages were scoped and a malignant growth was discovered. In a short period of time the cancer spread to his brain; death came quickly. He was in his forties when he died. It was hard to believe that Gordon, a big strong man, would die so young.

Bill Drew also passed on while still a young man. A businessman, he eventually became president of a trucking company that transported automobiles from the factory to their destination. We all owe him our thanks for introducing us to the lawyer who was instrumental in our acquisition of the land where the camp is situated.

Jim Blackwell, also deceased, lived two houses away from our home on Sylvan Avenue and later in the same condominium complex. He and his wife Matilda, nicknamed Tillie, were wonderful friends during our years as neighbours. Jim had a good singing voice and specialized in square dance music.

Two other former members, still alive, resigned from the camp for personal reasons. Our legal advisor, now a judge, was mentioned above. Clayton Hummel, a great guy and good friend, still lives in the Minden area. I still see these two gentlemen from time to time.

Our three guides, known as "doggers," were Harry Simmons, Al Reid, and Nat Pagnon. While not members, they came every year during the deer-hunting season. Their job was to walk through the bush making lots of noise so that the deer would move. Harry had served in the Korean War. In civilian life he was a real clown. He recounted lots of stories about the war; some of his stories may have even been true! In the bush, he always wore rubber hoots. He had a small farm where he raised pigs. Every year he said his female partner would have to clean the pigpens in her bare feet since he was wearing her boots in the bush!

Harry died from heart failure. Al and Nat are still associated with the camp and usually attend the annual Big Trout golf tournament.

In 2003 there were two resignations, Wilson Patterson and Roy Windover, both for personal reasons. Membership of the camp has been reduced to five. The long-term members include Keith Mountjoy, my college classmate, and Ken Giles who started the original group with me. More recent members include Don Woods, son of Barry Woods; Rick Mountjoy, son of Keith Mountjoy; and Dr. Peter Bennett, a fine young veterinarian who practises in Minden.

In 1993 the substantial physical activity that is a part of deer hunting became more than I could handle. Chest pain from severe angina was a regular daily occurrence. I decided that, since I was unable to do my share of the necessary camp work, it was time to tender my resignation. Several of the members said that they would be happy to do my share of the duties if I would reconsider. But my decision was final, and my resignation was accepted. I have made several return trips to the camp, always for a fishing expedition.

I have often wondered whether my participation at Big Trout Conservation Club, allowing me to get away from the stress of practice, may have been to the detriment of my family. Barbara looked after Janet while I enjoyed my days off in the bush. Who knows what might have happened if I had not had this stress release? A coronary thrombosis prior to age forty-nine?

As mentioned earlier, there were two camps within a short distance of each other on Big Trout Lake. Roy Windover's father had started the original camp on property sold to him by the Ontario government as a guide facility, used for the enjoyment of politicians. The property passed through several ownerships and was eventually purchased by a man named Glenn Kellett.

Glenn was good friend of mine for more than forty years. A farm boy raised in Haliburton County, he was, with his twin brother Craige, the last of a large family. Their parents had a difficult time financially. Glenn and Craige left school after completing grade eight. In spite of his lack of formal training, Glenn became the most successful entrepreneur I have ever known. He founded K-Line Maintenance and Construction Ltd. in 1967, a Canada-wide organization devoted to the transmission of electricity. This privately held company was later expanded to overseas operations in various countries. It eventually became the K-Line Group of Companies. One of the companies in this group manufactures electrical insulators. These were of superior quality to the old porcelain product. They were invented by Glenn and Craige and are now marketed throughout the world.

Each fall Glenn hosted a game dinner party and evening of country music at his cottage on Mountain Lake. The dinner consisted of various kinds of game and fish and usually concluded with wild-berry desserts. Usually no fewer than fifty people attended. Some of the guests brought their instruments. Glenn's favorite instrument was the mandolin. In spite of his huge fingers, he was very talented in producing music. Often he would temporarily exchange instruments with one of his brothers and continue playing without a hitch.

Glenn developed cancer of the pancreas, a disease normally fatal within six months. However he had an exceptional will to live and survived for two years from the date of diagnosis. After a valiant struggle with his malignancy, Glenn died on December 20, 2002. The following, previously written by Glenn, was included in the funeral service.

"Glenn's Values to Live By"

Always work hard and safely
Be positive
Be honest
Be innovative
Be prepared
Be independent
Be patient
Be understanding
Be genuine
Be modest
And
If music be the food of love,
Play on!

Glenn will be remembered as an avid outdoorsman with a common sense approach to life, an innovative spirit, a generous hospitality, a love of music, and a respect for nature. He will also be remembered for his approach to work and for his genuine concern for employees. I learned a lot about life from my good friend Glenn.

SECTION SEVEN

Breast Cancer

Chapter Thirty-Eight

Breast Cancer

Prior to our marriage, Barbara had surgery to remove a small cyst from one of her breasts, and several years later a second cyst was removed from the same breast. A cyst is a non-malignant fluid-filled sac and exhibits only mild discomfort. When palpated, a cyst yields to pressure almost as a grape might do if pressed. Barbara, as well as some others from of her nursing class, volunteered, shortly after graduation, to be part of a study group with respect to breast cancer. Each of the ladies in the group was asked to have an annual X-ray examination of her breasts to check for tumours. The study was conducted at the Woman's College Hospital in Toronto. They faithfully attended the hospital on an annual basis.

In 1985 she felt another abnormality in the same breast and without delay consulted our family physician. He decided that it was, in all probability, another cyst and should be of no concern. A few weeks later she asked me to examine the lump. I was very concerned, since it was hard and rather painful. I phoned the doctor, who was also a personal friend, and asked him to recheck the mass. He agreed that a biopsy should be done but still thought it was a cyst. When the biopsy proved positive for malignancy, an appointment was made with a surgeon. He gave us two options: radical mastectomy or lumpectomy. He recommended the radical mastectomy, explaining that in his experience it was the preferred method. We went home to digest this terrible news and to make a decision. My feeling was that the approach most likely to save her life was the one that should be undertaken. I was well aware that breast removal was likely to be mentally traumatic, but if it was the best way to accomplish survival then this approach should be undertaken. Barbara decided that since this was the best way to manage the problem, it should be done as soon as possible.

The mastectomy was completed within two weeks. Further bad news was forthcoming. We were told that when the pathologist examined the lymph nodes from under her arm, he discovered cancer cells. This indicated that the malignancy had already spread. Before her discharge from the hospital, an internal medicine specialist visited her to discuss the necessary post-operative treatment. Several approaches were explained— some relatively benign, others more aggressive. The one he wanted to use was a very aggressive procedure using a powerful drug that he said could cause severe reactions.

We were so overwhelmed with all of the bad news that we asked for some time to consider our options. I asked Janet, who had graduated in medicine, to do some research on the subject, and she was glad to consult with others and come up with some answers. I also asked a surgeon friend, Dr. Luke Teskey, a member of our hunting group, to check the literature and try to determine the best approach. Within a few days Janet and Luke had received replies from cancer specialists of four different Ontario teaching hospitals. Each was of the opinion that the aggressive treatment recommended by the internist was not indicated in this case. All suggested chemotherapy and radiation treatment as a preferable approach. I discussed this with the internist, who then recommended that we get an appointment at the Princess Margaret Hospital, a Toronto institution, specializing in the treatment of various types of cancer.

Since the malignancy had invaded the axillary lymph nodes, the oncologist at Princess Margaret recommended radiation of this area. They began a series of treatments. These completed, the next step was chemotherapy—a series of intravenous drugs whose purpose was the destruction of immature cells. Cancer cells are young cells that often grow rapidly and theoretically are subject to destruction by the toxic chemicals. Frequently as a side effect, young bone marrow cells may be destroyed at the same time, leading to anemia and other problems. In addition, the chemotherapy usually causes severe vomiting and, in many cases, loss of hair. It was distressing to see my poor wife undergo the ordeals of these various treatments that lasted for several months. In addition, an oral drug named tamoxifen was prescribed and was taken for several years. This drug was used in those cases of breast cancer related to the hormone estrogen. Theoretically, blocking the hormone controls the malignancy. In her case, it did not.

After the first year and the cessation of chemotherapy, Barbara to started to improve. She was able to play golf with her lady friends, as well as with me. We started to associate with our friends as soon as she felt comfortable in the company of others. Each winter we returned to Florida, usually to the Panhandle area. She again took an interest in investments, and it seemed as if her problem had been solved.

Since 1963 we had lived in a beautiful location on a hill overlooking Lake Ontario. While she was in remission, a new condominium development was proposed in our area. It seemed ideal for us to spend our retirement years here. We were among the first purchasers, long before construction began, and watched it being built. In spite of the building being finished, Barbara decided that she would like to stay in our home. The condominium was not occupied for two years.

For several years we assumed that her cancer was in remission.

For a Christmas present in 1990, I purchased a new set of golf clubs for her and put them under our tree. This pleased her, and she looked forward to using them, since we intended to leave for our winter trip in January. About the third time we played golf, she felt a severe pain on one side of the rib cage after swinging a club. We went to a local physician who ordered an X-ray examination of the affected area. To our dismay, the X-ray revealed a fractured rib. A metastatic tumour at the fracture site had eroded the bone to the point that the fracture easily occurred.

We stayed in Florida long enough for the weather to moderate in Canada and returned by mid-April. Upon our return, she went back to Princess Margaret for further therapy. She was admitted, then transferred to the Wellesley Hospital, next door to Princess Margaret, for her extended treatments. She was happy to be admitted to Wellesley, since she had graduated as a nurse from that hospital. Many of her classmates visited while she was hospitalized. This helped because her classmates were her best friends.

Janet and Michael's baby, Caroline, had been born the previous summer and was often brought to see her grandmother during the hospital stay. It pleased Barbara to see and to hold the child. She was well aware that this would be the only grandchild that she would know.

I closed my company, Multimed Realty, Inc., since I had little interest in working while my wife was in hospital. Each day I went to see her and tried to keep up her spirits. While the staff at the hospital kept encouraging us with respect to an optimistic prognosis, we both knew that recovery was very unlikely. Further X-ray examinations determined that the cancer had become more widespread and had extended to other bones. Early one morning, before my daily visit, the hospital called to advise me that she had fallen after getting out of a shower. She had a severe fracture of one of her femurs, again caused by a tumour eroding the bone. Orthopaedic surgery had to be done to repair the fracture, and the operation was done after midnight the next day. This was a terrible ordeal for a sick lady, but there was no other choice. I was annoyed that there had been no supervision when she had the shower and also because the mat that she stepped on after the shower was made of paper and was very slippery.

On several occasions we had discussed making charitable donations in our wills. We both agreed that the donations should be made to the Ontario Veterinary College, my alma mater, as well as to McMaster University where our daughter Janet had studied to achieve her degree in medicine. We both knew that there was a very limited amount of time left, so any financial decisions such as these donations were verified.

In late July we were told that she was terminal. She did not want to die in hospital and wanted to spend her final days in our home. Arrangements were made for the provision of twenty-four-hour-a-day nursing care in our home, and when that was arranged she came home by ambulance. Three nurses working on eight-hour shifts provided the care. The nurses were very professional and sympathetic with respect to our problem. By this time she was in so much pain that heavy doses of morphine, administered orally, were required to alleviate the discomfort.

One week later I felt that she would not last the night and asked Janet to come home to see her for the last time. When she saw her mother, she knew that the end was near. During the last night her nurses awakened me to advise me that she was not responding and that the pain was out of control. I decided that when the pharmacy opened the next morning I would acquire intravenous morphine and administer it myself to end her suffering. As a veterinarian I would not allow an animal to suffer in a like manner. Barbara died at 7:30 a.m., August 2, 1991, with Janet and me at her side. Had her death not occurred in this manner and had I proceeded, as was my intention, I would have notified the coroner. I have often wondered what the penalty would have been had this action taken place.

One of Janet's colleagues, Dr. Walter Himmel, came to our home to verify her death. This was most generous on his part since he had to cancel all of his office patients to make the house call. Later I chose him as my physician and found him to be outstanding in his field.

I was so drained emotionally that we decided to hold a private funeral service, for close relatives only, at the undertaker's establishment. Cremation, as per her request, followed the service. About three weeks later a memorial service was held at the Washington United Church, the church that we attended. Eulogies were given by Nora Clark, one of Barbara's nursing friends, and by Roly Armitage, who had been best man at our wedding more than forty years earlier. Many friends and acquaintances attended the memorial service, another difficult day for me.

Two months after her death, I decided to move from the house to our condominium that had been available but not used for two years. I had to find a tenant for the house, since the real estate market was difficult and house prices had dropped substantially. About two years elapsed between the first tenant and the eventual sale. The first tenant, a young golf professional from our club, was ideal. He had to be replaced after accepting a new post in British Columbia. The next tenant, a young bachelor and also a golf pro, had numerous drinking parties and was less than satisfactory. He had to be evicted. The place was unfit for showing to potential purchasers during his stay.

The move required the purchase of new appliances as well as some furniture. Not familiar with decorating ideas, I enlisted the help of some good friends, Dr. and Mrs. Jim Lennox, of Barrie. Jim had been a classmate of mine. They often visited Barbara during her stay in hospital; Barbara had asked Marian to help me when she was no longer with us. Their assistance was invaluable during this transitional period.

During the first month at the new residence, many letters of appreciation had to be written to those who had been helpful during the difficult period. Many floral tributes had been sent, as well as donations made to a variety of charitable organizations. I had not realized what an emotional experience it could be to write so many thank-you letters.

Later Years

Chapter Thirty-Nine

September Romance

In September, 1991, I accepted with pleasure an invitation to a salmon fishing trip in Campbell River, British Columbia. Several of those on the trip were men I had met previously. We had a great experience and caught plenty of Coho salmon.

A golfing friend, Wally Lord, had also lost his wife the same summer. A group of golf members from our club had booked a November week of golf at a resort near Orlando, Florida. Wally was one of those in the group. He and I had a number of discussions about a winter trip and decided to drive to Florida to spend the month of March, 1992. It was good to join up for these trips since we had so much in common.

In May of 1992, Owen Grimbly, who leased the condominium next door to mine, asked me if I would join him as well as his sister and another lady for dinner in his unit, to be followed by a game of bridge, the arrival time to be 5:30 in the afternoon. I accepted.

Every fifteen minutes between 5:30 and 6:30, I knocked on his door with no response. Between these attempts, I would go back to my unit and sip on a scotch. Eventually they arrived and he introduced his sister to me as Joan (no last name was given). Apparently Joan perceived the odour of scotch and commented to her brother that his next-door neighbour must be a lush.

When it came time to cook the dinner (a sirloin steak), Owen confessed to his sister and the other lady that making the dinner was beyond his culinary expertise, and would they take over the kitchen duties? They agreed, and eventually the meal was served. The bridge game followed, and Owens's ability at the bridge table was a substantial improvement over his expertise in the kitchen.

A week or so later I returned the dinner invitation to the same group. There was some venison in my freezer from the previous year's deer hunting expedition, and I put it on the menu. I made it quite clear to the guests that, unlike the last dinner party, assistance of the ladies in the kitchen would not be necessary.

The next morning I had a phone call from some lady named Joan.

"Joan who?" I asked.

"Joan Lounsbury, the lady you had dinner with last night." Since Owen had not given her a last name at the introduction, she forgave me.

Two weeks later Joan phoned again and suggested a bridge weekend at her cottage on Lake Rosseau. I accepted. Lake Rosseau is a two-and-a-half-hour trip by car, north and west of Toronto. Since her cottage was on an island, called Ouno Island, it was necessary for her to pick up guests by boat from the car parking area. The boat trip took about ten minutes. She recited a history of the property. The grand old cottage, a large structure with several outbuildings, had been built in 1897. One of the boathouses is a landmark on the lake because of an unusual feature. The original owner had a great interest in sailboats and had the building housing one of them especially designed to permit entry of the thirty-five-foot-high mast.

The cottage was quite impressive in size and appearance. The walls were all wood, panelled with lumber of that era, no longer available. Six bedrooms available in the main cottage could house large numbers of guests. Some of the outbuildings provided additional sleeping accommodation. The lot, with some 1500 feet of shoreline, offered good southern exposure. A retired man did general property maintenance on a part-time basis.

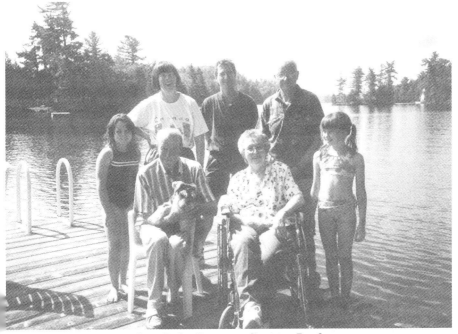

Our Lake Rosseau Cottage Dock
Back Row: Janet Graham, Michael Tarjan, Bob Green
Front Row: Suzanne (Caroline's friend), Blake Graham,
Margaret Green, Caroline Tarjan

Joan and I talked a lot during this visit. She had been married early in life and had three children from the marriage. Her husband died as the result of a massive coronary at forty-two years of age. The youngest child, John, was only four years old when his father died. Later Joan married again, this time to an engineer named Ian Lounsbury who had one child named Roger. Roger's mother had died of breast cancer. After some years of marriage, Joan and Ian decided by mutual agreement to obtain a legal separation. Joan had been unattached for several years prior to our meeting. She also told me that Ian was now suffering from malignant melanoma and had been told that it was incurable.

I told Joan that I was still mourning the loss of my wife and that my life seemed to lack direction. She was very sympathetic with respect to my problems. The fact that she had experienced the same thing made it easier for her to understand.

On the drive back to the city the next day, I thought a lot about Joan and felt that our meeting was fortunate. She seemed to be a delightful lady, well read as the result of her university background in literature, very attractive, and in general exhibiting good humour. Although Barbara had been gone less than a year, I felt that it was time to change my disconsolate attitude. My mind was made up to see this lady again.

We had a few dates in the city before the next visit to her cottage. This time she had a large family group in residence. Her daughter Nancy and son-in-law Jim Wilson had three daughters—Maxine, Adrienne, and Carolyn. Nancy and her daughters spent most of the summer season at the cottage with Jim visiting on weekends. I was made welcome by the group and enjoyed the weekend with them. On the next visit to the cottage, I met her son John, a fine young man whose company I enjoyed. It was some months later before I met her oldest son Charlie, since he rarely visited the cottage.

That summer we had two large parties on Ouno Island. The old flagstaff had fallen and had to be replaced. The replacement necessitated its transportation by barge and required the skills of several local men to put in position. Joan decided that it would be appropriate, in honour of the 125th anniversary of

Canada, to have a luncheon followed by the flag raising ceremony. Many of her friends, including several families who were cottage neighbours and who arrived in their own boats, joined the party. Among the guests was one of her friends from public school, Evangeline (Vange) Croucher, as well as Vange's husband Jack. Since this was to be my first meeting with Vange and Jack, I hoped to pass inspection! Jack and Joan's granddaughter Maxine delivered a rousing rendition of "Oh Canada" in French.

Later in the summer we had a dinner party that included a lot of my friends and some of Joan's. My outdoor friends, accomplished in the art of country music, played bluegrass, the theme music of the party. In the late afternoon a group of the musicians boarded boats and, with their motors at slow speed, toured the area playing their instruments. Several of our boats followed the fiddlers and guitar players. Neighbouring cottagers went to their docks to see the flotilla and gave ringing applause. The musicians returned to the cottage and continued playing on the expansive cottage verandas, much to the delight of the other guests. Those unable to play an instrument joined in singing some of the old favourites. A buffet dinner was served, after which the music continued to the wee hours. Most of the guests could be provided sleeping accommodation, some being allocated chesterfields. After breakfast the next morning, the guests, no doubt a few with thick heads, departed.

Janet and my sister Margaret began to wonder why I was not answering the telephone. I told them I was dating a lady and that introductions would soon take place. When Janet was introduced to Joan, they seemed to enjoy the company of each other. Of course this was important to me. In the latter part of the summer, Joan, as well as a group of her female friends, went on a two-week trip to Germany. She had always enjoyed travelling and had been to many places around the world. I missed her company while she was away and was very pleased to see her return.

Vange and Jack were at both of our parties. Presumably I must have passed inspection, since Joan and I were invited to visit their cottage near Minden. They spent their winter months in Florida at a place called Anna Maria Island. Joan had visited Anna Maria on a previous occasion and had found it to be pleasant, and free from the honky-tonk atmosphere that exists in some southern communities. We decided that perhaps a winter together would give us a good indication as to the potential permanence of our relationship. We asked Vange to investigate the area to find a suitable rental unit for the winter. She found one situated on the Gulf of Mexico near the Croucher's accommodation. This house, owned by the famous baseball player Warren Spahn, was named, appropriately, Home Plate.

Jack Croucher had enlisted with the navy and served during the Second World War, based in Halifax. He told me the following story and as it has something to do with animals, I thought it would be proper to include it in this narrative. It is a true story. I entitled his account "Mounties as Diagnosticians."

Jack was a junior officer in the RCNVR at the beginning of the Second World War. Because of a shortage of housing, many new trainees were billeted in Halifax, a short ferry ride from the naval base in Dartmouth. Jack and several of his naval buddies had sleeping quarters in a private home in Halifax. Other occupants of the house included the owners, a young married couple, their small child, and their friendly female golden retriever.

After a late evening at the local pub, Jack and his buddies made their way back to their rooms, a fifteen-minute walk through heavy rain. Rather than search for the clothes closet in the dark, Jack decided to leave his new Burberry raincoat draped over the hat stand in the vestibule. He failed to notice that the coat had slid off the arm of the hat stand and landed partly on the seat and partly on the floor.

The young sailors had to leave their rooms well before daylight in order to catch the first ferry to Dartmouth. It became obvious as they reached the lights of the ferry dock that they were being pursued by a motley group of curs of all sizes and colours. The beasts complained mournfully when they were not allowed to accompany the lads aboard the ferry.

At lunch break the young sailors decided that a wee tot at the pub might help alleviate their cranial discomfort, the result of their indiscretions of the previous evening. To get to the pub they had to go through a gate to the ferry guarded by two RCMP officers in full uniform, their red coats resplendent in the noonday sunshine. On the way to the pub they were again accompanied by the parade of dogs that had patiently waited for the sailors. After the liquid fortification the men returned to the ferry gate, followed by the dogs. One of the Mounties asked Jack if by any chance he might be related to the Pied Piper. Jack replied that he had no explanation for the canine escort. The other Mountie, who prided himself as a consummate detective, was not amused by the appearance of the sailors and commented, "By your bloodshot eyes and the smell of stale beer, it is obvious that you lads have been drinking too much. Your Burberry coat is a disgrace, since it is damp, wrinkled, and covered with hair from a dog. By the colour and size of the hair, it came from a golden retriever, and by the attention being paid to your coat by this pack of male dogs, it should have been obvious, even to a bunch of beer drinkers like you guys, that the retriever slept on your coat and left the canine perfume of a bitch in heat."

Jack passed away after a long battle with a chronic illness. His self-deprecating humour will always be remembered.

Our winter was pleasant, and the relationship between Joan and me matured. We delighted in the company of each other. Through the Crouchers we met a lot of other people, some of whom were Canadian.

We spent the summer of 1993 at Joan's cottage. Since it was old, the place required substantial maintenance; it was very large and expensive for her to maintain. She decided to sell the big cottage, and we looked for a smaller property on the same lake. We found a buyer who was charmed with Ouno and its history. We found another cottage, also on an island, again a most attractive cottage. Together we purchased it. I bought a pontoon boat with a capacity of twelve, ideal for our use. The boathouse on this property had a slip wide enough for the new boat, as well as one for Joan's boat. The boathouse had a second story with a delightful one-bedroom apartment facing south, with an excellent view overlooking the lake. Our guests used this apartment.

During the summer of 1994, we felt that we were compatible and very fond of each other. I decided to propose marriage to Joan, who gracefully accepted. Barbara and I had, on different occasions over the years, discussed the possibility of death. We had agreed that whichever survived should not live a life of abstinence and should find another companion. Joan's son John and his fiancée Shirley were to be married that year, so we set our wedding date for November 12, 1994. The wedding was a small affair, family only, held in Joan's home. We decided to do things a little differently from the normal and had John act as Joan's bridesmaid and I had Janet act as my best man. This reversal of roles lasted only to the conclusion of the ceremony! Joan's brother Owen gave the toast to the bride and in his speech noted that "Blake likes to cook and Joan likes to eat, so it should make for a harmonious relationship."

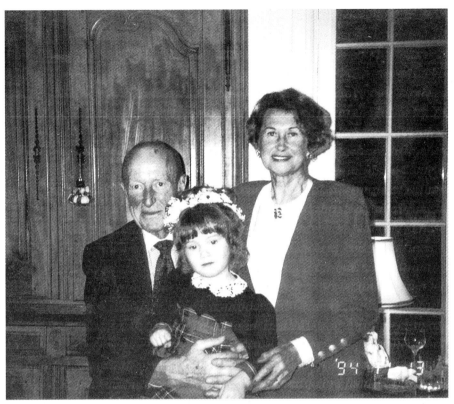

Blake and Joan's Wedding Day:
Blake, Joan, Caroline

Chapter Forty

The Barbara Graham Breast Cancer Research Fund

Barbara and I had decided to make contributions to the Ontario Veterinary College and to McMaster University. Instructions were contained in our wills. After her death, it seemed that there was nothing to be gained by waiting until after mine to begin a research program and that investigation into suitable projects should be started. I contacted the two teaching institutions and advised them of my intentions. I asked for a joint meeting, with the instructions that proposals should be made for my consideration. The first meeting was held in 1993 at McMaster University in Hamilton. A variety of potential projects were tabled.

This was my first meeting with Dr. Jack Gauldie, Chairman, Department of Pathology and Director, Immunology Laboratory, McMaster University. One of Dr. Gauldie's cancer research projects involving mice fascinated me. The mice were injected with human breast cancer cells that survived and grew to be large tumours in the mice. Some of the cancer tissue was then removed from the mice, and their genetic components were modified in his laboratory. The changed genes were then covered with human adenovirus that acted as a transport medium when injected back to the mice. The immune system of the mice attacked the modified genes as well as the original cancer cells to which the modified genes had become attached. He showed photographs of the mice before and after treatment. In most cases there was substantial reduction in the size of the tumours. Some of the mice had multiple tumours, and when the genetically modified cancer cells were introduced at one site, reduction in the size of some of the other tumours was observed. This indicated that the modified genetic material, rather than being confined to one site, had been conveyed to the other sites. This was an important finding in that breast cancer, in many cases, metastasizes to other areas of the body.

After a few days of considering this research as well as the other projects submitted, I felt that Dr. Gauldie's project would be worthy of support. I found out a few days later that the London Life Insurance Company had also made a donation of $300,000.00 to this same project because they were aware of Dr. Gauldie's exceptional research capabilities. The two original donations were combined as start-up money for this project. One stipulation that I had made was that the two universities, the Ontario Veterinary College and McMaster, should work together. Dr. Gauldie welcomed this co-operation and began discussions with Dr. Steve Kruth from Guelph, who had attended the first meeting. The co-operation between the two organizations has been outstanding, and each has made contributions that added to the research project. I was aware that this was a long-term project, would require a lot of money, and there was no guarantee of success. Even if a project does not fulfill expectations, it provides a base for further study in the same field and could be important to medicine.

In Barbara's memory the project was named the Barbara Graham Breast Cancer Research Fund. It was my hope that this research would lead to a better understanding of, and possibly a better treatment for, this disastrous disease.

In 1994 I wrote letters to friends and colleagues in my profession, as well as to other friends. The letter discussed my role in this new project and asked for donations to be used for the research. Many donations were forthcoming, with both universities receiving funds. An official publication of the Ontario Veterinary College called *The Crest* is sent to all graduates of the Ontario Veterinary College. The publication dated December, 1994 contained the following article:

Dr. Blake Graham, an OVC 1951 graduate and retired veterinarian, has made an extraordinary pledge to the Ontario Veterinary College and to McMaster University—$200,000.00 to each institution for co-operative research on cancer. Specifically they will be investigating the merits of cytokine gene transfer as it relates to cancer in dogs and humans.

OVC's team, that will be studying cancer in dogs, consists of Dr. Steve Kruth, clinical studies, and Anne Croy, Allan King and Jon LaMarre. McMaster's team studying human breast cancer includes Dr. Jack Gauldie, Professor and Chair, Department of Pathology/Director Immunology Laboratory and another OVC graduate Dr. Ron Carter, OVC 1983, also from McMaster's Department of Pathology.

Dr. Graham and his daughter, Dr. Janet Graham, visited OVC November 10 for a planning meeting that included representatives from McMaster and Guelph. During lunch he presented the next instalment of his commitment—$61,000.00 each to Guelph president Dr. Mordechai Rodanski and to Dr. Gauldie. (Some months ago he made an initial donation to the Guelph project of over $71,000.00, the first to be channelled through the university's new Crown agency, with an identical donation to McMaster).

Dr. Graham has always felt grateful to OVC for his professional training. This led, he claimed, to his being "reasonably successful in veterinary practice" so that he was able to invest a small amount of money each year in order to build up a capital base. He feels equally grateful to McMaster where his only daughter Janet received her medical training. "So," he said, "I feel I owe something to both institutions."

His main incentive, however, was to find an appropriate memorial for his late wife, Barbara, who died of breast cancer. He considers horrendous the treatment she had to undergo. It reminds him of the time when he was an undergraduate at OVC and observed "firing," a treatment then used for lameness in horses. "We have to find a better way of treating breast cancer," he stated.

Both teams will use a strategy of isolating malignant cells, infecting them with a virus containing genes that are expected to make the cancer cells better targets for destruction by the animal's or person's own immune system, then giving the cells back to the patient.

"Cancer in pets has always been a relatively common problem," says Dr. Kruth. "In the past the animal was usually euthanized as soon as the diagnosis was made, but over the past twenty years owner attitudes have changed; pets are now seen as true family members; owners have a better understanding of what's possible in therapy so veterinarians are called on more frequently to treat these animals."

Further donations to the research project resulted from this publication. As the research project progressed, both universities found that the start-up funding had become exhausted. Minor donations came in, but not enough to fund the work adequately. One large drug company wanted to fund the program for several million dollars, but when it found that this method of therapy in all probability could not be patented, the company declined to participate. Various other methods of funding were attempted and met with some success. Subsequently, major funding came from donations to McMaster made by graduates of the institution, with some of these funds being directed to our project. In addition, some funding came from government and other sources.

On February 20, 2002, I sent this e-mail to Drs. Gauldie and Kruth:

Dear Jack and Steve:

I am in the process of writing the story of my life. The title will be "Anecdotes from the Life of a Veterinarian." Included will be a chapter on breast cancer. It would be much appreciated if both of you would provide me with the current status of the Barbara Graham Breast Cancer Research Project. In particular I wish to include whether or not there is a reasonable chance of the project having a long-term benefit for those people suffering from the disease. In addition, is the project likely to have any benefit for the management of other forms of malignancy? Best regards to both...

The following were the replies from Dr. Gauldie, dated February 20, 2002, and from Dr. Kruth, dated February 22, 2002:

Blake:

I will look forward to having an opportunity to read about the history of an unusual individual!! As regards to the question about where we are regarding breast cancer, we have just concluded the writing of a proposal to Health Protection Branch Canada to embark on the first clinical trial in Canada (and probably the world) aimed at using gene therapy to stimulate the immune response against a specific marker on breast cancer cells with a cell-based gene vaccine approach. This is based on a series of pre-clinical studies that started with the work supported by the Barbara Graham Fund and has taken

274

us all the way to this exciting clinical trial. We expect to get to the clinical trial sometime towards the end of the year after we get the material produced at a clinical grade level and have permission from HPB to proceed. The start-up support you provided has grown into significant support from CIHR, NCIC and CAN VAC, the Canadian Centre of Excellence in immunotherapy and infectious disease. You can be proud that the first investment you made has now allowed major initiatives in the development of gene-based immunotherapy for breast cancer. I would be pleased to provide more details as we go on and have you visit with us to meet the clinicians involved in the trial. Let me know your wishes

— Jack

Hi Blake,

Glad to hear from you. I hope that you are having a good winter in Florida. The weather here certainly was not consistent with weather in Ontario. I am very glad that you are writing an autobiography. It is difficult to find real role models for young veterinary students, and I feel that your life story will be both inspiring and instructive. I am looking forward to reading it, so please let me know when it comes available.

The Barbara Graham Trust is very active at OVC. As you know, as it turns out that canine breast cancer per se is not a great animal model for the human condition, so we looked for alternatives, namely osteosarcoma and melanoma. We supplied these models to Dr. Gauldie to assist his group in developing anti-cancer vaccines in general. His group has used that knowledge to find alternative and effective methods of treating human breast cancer as well as other cancers. One of the beauties of this mode of cancer therapy is that it is a general tool with the potential of being targeted to not only specific cancer (e.g.

breast cancer, osteosarcoma, melanoma etc) but to the individual's specific cancer within that general type.

We know that your primary intent was to move human therapy forward, and I believe that our group has contributed to that goal. However we are also developing the same therapies for veterinary patients. We are just completing a clinical trial of gene therapy in cats with cancer, with good results. Again this feeds back into treatment for humans to some degree.

One of the really important things is that your support allowed us to establish a laboratory dedicated to the study of animal models of cancer. These facilities were the beginning of several collaborations using dogs, cats and other animals as models for human disease. Your initial vision allowed us to expand, and a few of us at OVC wrote a proposal to the Canadian Foundation for Innovation entitled *Institute for Animal-Human Links in the Study of Disease*. We were just notified that we were completely successful to the tune of $27.5 million plus change. We will be building this facility over the next few years. It is really important to know that you initiated this idea, that your support allowed it to grow, and that without your support and vision it would never have happened.

The animal modeling will ultimately support cancer therapy in humans (again spinning back to the treatment of breast cancer among others)—it will support research in other areas too, especially in arthritis. We have just become a research centre for the Canadian Arthritis Network, which is a Canadian Centre of Excellence. In summary, your support at OVC did not lead to a direct development in human breast cancer therapy. It did lead to more general models that we believe were and continue to be useful to Dr. Gauldie's group. We have moved forward in veterinary medicine. We now have a facility on the horizon that is designed to *support comparative medicine, including cancer therapy research (with spins that will alter how women with breast cancer are managed. A circuitous route, but nevertheless very beneficial for humans and animals).*

Best Wishes,
Stephen

I was elated to read these e-mails as at long last there appeared to be the possibility of major breakthroughs in the management of some types of cancer. I will be accepting Jack's invitation to have a personal look at his work and to congratulate his great team on their achievements. Janet and I are delighted to have played a minor role in this research project, should it prove to be a benefit in the future to women suffering from breast cancer. Even if it does not meet all of our hopes for reducing deaths from human breast cancer, the effort was worthwhile and we know that we made the correct decision. In addition, the work being done at OVC has aided the McMaster studies and will, when their new facilities are in operation, be a major step forward in assisting future research that will benefit both animals and man. This project was conceived with the idea of starting co-operation between the two universities for long-range studies in comparative medicine and perhaps in other areas of research. It appears that this will happen.

On the morning of September 11, 2002, I received the following e-mail from Dr. Gauldie. I was delighted with his progress in the research and with the help of the dedicated, excellent team of research staff. Not only is major progress being made in potential breast cancer therapy, but other types of malignancies are being studied and these other types of cancer may also show response to his unique therapy. I look forward to meeting his group to express my thanks for their outstanding work.

Blake:

My apologies for the slowness of the reply. This is the heaviest time for new grants, and I have another one due September 15. I have been trying to get some time set aside to have you meet with the people running the trial here in Hamilton. It looks like the best time to get together will be the first week in November, as we are away at a meeting on vaccines and gene therapy during the last part of September. If you mean that you could be here the last two weeks in October, that would also be good.

I have only good news to report to you about the breast vaccine trial. We have started the process of producing the vaccine at a pharmaceutical grade ready for human use. This is a big undertaking and costs us $220,000.00 US for a lot to treat up to twenty-five patients. We have already obtained one grant for $125,000.00 CDN from the province and yesterday heard that we have been selected for a competition for funding from the Canadian Breast Cancer Research Initiative. This grant, if we are success-ful, should fund the entire trial over the next three years. (I always seem to be writing grants.)

Our results with skin cancer gene vaccine are very encouraging, and we expect the same progress will occur when we start the breast trial in early 2003. I hope that we can get together and you can meet this young group of clin-icians who are putting to practise the things that we first developed with your support. Let me know if the November date is good and I will set up a lunch for us to meet with the others. It would be good to have a chance to meet with Colin Brown as well. I can let you see the plans for the new research building going up behind the hospital to house our research activity. We got some of the funding from the Feds and others from the province. The university foots the rest, and they are now on the fundraising trail. We got the funds because we had made such progress in establishing *the gene vaccine approach. So your support does not stop at providing research activities; we have parlayed it well beyond our earlier dreams. Our research-building project is now worth $30 million. Not a bad investment!!*

Best regards,
Jack.

I received another helping of encouraging news as I approached conclusion of this book. On December 15, 2003, Steve Kruth wrote, with regard to progress:

Specifically, the gene therapy project with Dr. Gauldie is heating up. I just entered a new dog with oral melanoma this past week, and Dr. Gauldie's lab currently is doing the gene transfer. Due to a reorganization of my resources, I expect to enrol several dogs within the next few months. This is very exciting work, as we are developing the new dendritic cell based gene transfer technique. We presented our research at an international meeting in the States last month. I would be happy to provide more details if you need it.

Steve had some exciting news about the Institute for Animal-Human Links in the Study of Disease as well:

The new research building is designed to facilitate the use of non-rodent animal models. Some of the research will be that of individual OVC faculty members, but the majority will be collaborative work between OVC faculty and investigators at medical schools or from industry. I expect to see a large number of projects in the areas of gene therapy, cancer, neurology, cardiovascular disease, and orthopedic surgery. New therapies, including gene therapy and surgical interventions, as well as drug development will be targeted. The outcomes will benefit human medicine primarily, with lots of secondary benefit for veterinary species. The new building will con-

*tain surgeries, an intensive care facility, short-term hous-
ing, imaging facilities, ultrasound, etc.*

*The ground should be broken this spring, with a two-
year timeline to opening. The cost is 3.5 M construction,
with another 3.5 M for equipment.*

*The same CFI grant funded our new MRI unit.
That building has started, with the unit opening this
coming August.*

There was even an offer of a job:

*Unfortunately, after a year-long international
search, we have not been able to find a new hospital
director (are you looking for a new challenge?)*

...to which I replied:

*I am honoured that you have asked me to consider
accepting a position at OVC, however I must decline
because of old age!*

The December 18, 2003 edition of *The Hamilton Spectator*
carried this startling headline:

MAC MEDICAL SCHOOL GIVEN $105 MILLION

This astonishing donation, the biggest individual donation
in Canadian history, covered the university's entire objective
for 2003. It was the gift of businessman and philanthropist
Michael G. DeGroote, apparently following a conference with
some of his family. The *Spectator* quoted Mr. DeGroote: "This
gift is intended to support health-care research and education...I am investing in new discoveries in health care and the
delivery of health care...the dividends of that investment will
not only impact our community, but others around the world."
I phoned Peter George, president of McMaster, who assured me
that a lot of this money will be devoted to cancer research with
a good amount directed to Jack Gauldie's project; it will be a
great boost to the Barbara Fund.

Chapter Forty-One

Change of Address

The charming small cottage on Lake Rosseau had a disadvantage. When I began to have severe angina, I realized that the island location would make it difficult to obtain medical treatment in the event of a cardiac emergency. We received an unsolicited offer for this cottage, and we accepted it. After a period of searching for another cottage, we found an old farmhouse on the mainland that met our requirements and negotiated a successful purchase. This cottage was adequate for all of the family on both sides since it had six bedrooms and had the added advantage that no major repairs were necessary. We sold this property in November 2002 and purchased another cottage at Southampton, Ontario. This property, close to the village, is on the shore of Lake Huron. Southampton is a lovely town. The residents are very friendly; invariably they wish you "good morning" when you meet on the street. Southampton advertises itself as having "the best sunsets in Canada." Each evening during the summer, the sight of the sun disappearing into the water of Lake Huron is magnificent.

After our marriage Joan and I changed residence several times. I sold the condominium in Scarborough and moved to her home on Lonsdale Road in mid Toronto where we lived with John and Shirley, his new wife. This house was too small for four people. We found a three-story residence for sale on Heath Street in the Yonge and St. Clair area of Toronto and purchased it. Extensive renovations were necessary prior to the move. Joan and I took over the first floor, John and Shirley the second floor, and Joan's brother Owen took over the top floor. This new house was ideal for us, since we spent most of the summers at the cottage and most of the winters in Florida. Having someone look after the residence during our absence presented us a major advantage. Soon after we moved to Heath Street, my problem with angina worsened. I made an appointment for cardiac catheterization at the Hamilton General Hospital. Four of the arteries to the left ventricle were substantially blocked, and immediate surgery was necessary. Fortunately the tests were done a few days before Christmas and the cardiac surgeon was able to fit me in very quickly. Four vessels were bypassed, and the recovery was uneventful.

Florida appealed to us so much that we decided rather than rent winter accommodation we should purchase a home on Anna Maria Island. We purchased a condominium unit in a very quiet area, occupied mainly by snowbirds from the States and from Canada, with a few year-round residents. We occupied it for two years. Another unit in the same complex came up for sale. This unit overlooks the inland waterway and has a pretty view. Neglected two years, it needed extensive renovations. We upgraded, and it is now our pleasant place to spend the winter months.

Retrospections and Observations

Chapter Forty-Two

Foot and Mouth Disease

*As these memoirs draw to a close, I look back on
a few episodes and reflections seemingly sub-
merged in the past. They are, nonetheless,
linked to the present and the future and therefore require attention.*

In December of 1951, while we were in California, I received
a letter from a classmate, Dr Harold Hunter, who had started a
practice in Regina, Saskatchewan. In his letter Harold
described an outbreak of disease on a farm in his area. He was
convinced that the disease was foot-and-mouth disease, a
highly infectious disease of cloven-footed animals. Endemic in
Europe, the disease had never been reported in Canada. At college it had been described in our studies, but since it was not a
problem in our part of the world we had never seen a clinical
case. The disease manifests itself by blisters in the mouth and
the feet of infected animals, accompanied by weight loss due to

inability to eat. Harold reported his findings to the Federal Department of Agriculture as well as to the Saskatchewan Department of Agriculture. Both government agencies disputed the diagnosis. They believed the disease to be vesicular stomatitis, which has some similarities from a symptomatic point of view, is much less severe, and is unlikely to cripple the livestock industry. Harold stood by his convictions and insisted on laboratory examinations to either confirm or reject his opinion.

At that time federal regulations prohibited the transport of infected animal tissues out of the province. On February 14, 1952, Dr. Carlson, a provincial veterinarian in Regina, against federal regulations sent the infected tissues to the federal laboratory in Hull, Quebec, for analysis. The diagnosis of foot-and-mouth disease was confirmed on February 25. This confirmation came some three months after Dr. Hunter's original clinical diagnosis. Now drastic steps had to be taken in order to control the further spread of the disease. The farm where it was first diagnosed, as well as the other farms to which it had spread, became subject to strict quarantine. All of the cattle, sheep and hogs on these farms were slaughtered then buried in deep pits, covered with lime, and buried with soil.

Diagnosis confirmed, an army of federal veterinarians arrived in Saskatchewan to inspect the farms in the area and to institute disinfection procedures on the affected farms. It would be fair to say that the time loss between the tentative diagnosis and the final diagnosis cost the taxpayers of Canada many millions. This loss included the destruction of some 4,000 animals. In his article "Marked for Death" in *Western People,* James Whalen quotes then Federal Minister of Finance Douglas Abbott as telling Parliament "the total loss on hogs and cattle related to foot-and-mouth disease was just over $69 million." According to the Internet Inflation Calculator of S. Morgan Friedman, that would amount to $459,800,853.00 in the year 2002. Had the clinical diagnosis been accepted, or at least investigated, and laboratory confirmation made at that time, the losses would have been confined to the original farm with a substantial reduction in cost to the Canadian taxpayers.

An amusing instance of federal government inefficiency arises in this little vignette from the memoirs of Norman Wagner, President Emeritus of the University of Calgary, offered in a poignant Internet article entitled "Foot-and-Mouth Disease—A Regina Teenager's Memories."

We were allowed to keep them (the chickens) for a very short while. What struck me as almost comical was the directive that the eggs too might be contaminated. We dumped them in piles in the yard, and as the snow came, the mound of dangerous eggs grew larger. Don't ask what it was like in the spring.

To those who have to feed them, chickens are best described as "ankle peckers." This was the time when chickens roamed rather freely and you had to walk among them. I must say I didn't miss them, but I'm sure that if one had a pet chicken the feeling would be different. Five thousand is just too big a mob to begin to love one at a time.

My dad struck a blow for the cause of farming when he negotiated with a government man…The poor sod had never been on a farm. His naive question, "How many eggs will a chicken lay in a day?" brought a wry smile to my dad's face. He suggested that two might be a fair number, seven days a week. He could have asked for more, but he knew the limit. And, some chickens do manage two eggs a day!

The math was straightforward. Two times five thousand times 365 times the going price was the compensation agreed upon. The government man even offered to pay for all the feed they might have eaten, since we no doubt had purchased it in advance! Oh yes, all hay and straw had to go as well. The farm was stripped of all

*life and feed. Despite the sorrow, this is one year we
made money farming!*

An article in the *Globe and Mail* of March 15, 2001, by
Dawn Walton was entitled "Virus (Foot-and-Mouth Virus)
Came to Canada with a Migrant Farm Worker." She related
how a German migrant worker named Willi Bruntjen came to
Canada carrying dried sausage in his baggage. He had come
from Germany where, at that time, foot-and-mouth disease was
endemic. He worked on the original farm for only a few days
before leaving for a larger farming operation. He left wearing
the same overalls. Three explanations exist with respect to the
transmission of the virus by the farm worker. He may have fed
some of the sausage to the farm dogs that in turn defecated in
the barnyard, depositing the virus. He may have thrown some
of the sausage in the watering tank used by the cattle, or he
may have used the barnyard for his own depository. The precise
method of transmission is unimportant. Most importantly, Ms.
Walton noted how quickly the virus can spread and how one
person can unwittingly cripple the entire agricultural economy.
She failed to note that Dr. Hunter had made the original diagnosis and that it was not accepted by his peers.

An article by Krista Foss in the same newspaper dated
March 21, 2001, was entitled "How the Mounties Saved the
Canadian Beef Industry." In it she highlighted how the Mounties
shot the animals and described the macabre aspect of the butch-
ers eviscerating the livestock to prevent the odours of decompo-
sition. Like Walton she failed to mention the role of Dr. Hunter,
who by himself made the original diagnosis of the problem.

In my opinion, Dr. Hunter had made the most important
diagnosis in the history of Canadian veterinary medicine. I
took exception to the inaccuracies of these articles, particularly
those of Ms. Foss, and expressed my opinion by e-mail. Her
reply was that she had three articles for the paper that day and
had not considered the facts of the case beyond the interview

with a retired Mountie who had been involved in the destruction of the infected animals, victims of the outbreak.

Dr. Hunter, who had been a roommate of mine during our college years, died many years ago after a long battle with cancer. I also knew his wife June, whom he married soon after graduation. It seemed to me that an important milestone in veterinary medicine was missing and that it should be rectified. I was not sure (and am still not convinced) whether this was a deliberate or an accidental loss of veterinary history. The 50th anniversary of our graduation was to occur in June of 2001. I decided to pursue the matter to see if the government of Canada could give recognition to his widow at our anniversary celebration.

I started a letter-writing campaign, with letters to Mr. Lyle Vanclief, Minister of Agriculture, as well as various Members of Parliament. There was little interest in my letters, so I started to phone various contacts in the Department of Agriculture in Ottawa. I was told that there were no records of Dr. Hunter having any participation in the outbreak. I advised them to contact the newspapers, in particular the *Regina Leader Post* and the *Guelph Mercury*, which had articles on the problem at the time of the outbreak, and that these articles were available in their archives. The articles specifically identified Dr. Hunter's role in the outbreak. When these sources of information were given to the department, there appeared to have been a change in their attitude.

I enlisted the support of Dr. Meek, Dean of the Ontario Veterinary College, to put some pressure on the Department of Agriculture. Eventually a letter from Dr. Brian Evans, Chief Veterinary Officer for Canada, was received and read at our anniversary.

Excerpts from his letter stated that the members of the Class of OVC 51 have each made their own contribution to the legacy of excellence in animal health and food safety, for which both the profession and the Canadian public owe a debt of gratitude.

Recent public interest in foot-and-mouth disease arising from the current outbreaks in Europe and South America has highlighted the critical role played by Dr. Hunter of the class of 51 in the early diagnosis and containment of the only occurrence of the disease in Canada: Saskatchewan, 1952. The original clinical diagnosis was made in December, 1951, and its confirmation by laboratory tests was made on February 25, 1952. Neither Doctor Evans nor Mr. Vanclief has cited this disastrous loss of precious time.

Dr. Hunter's efforts and perseverance speak to the seamless and synergistic relationships that are necessary between all interested parties and bear strong testament to the reality that most successful outcomes start with the commitment of an individual.

A few weeks after our 50th anniversary celebration, June Hunter received a letter from Mr. Vanclief, Minister of Agriculture, in which he recognized that her late husband was in fact the veterinarian who had made the original diagnosis. He had several months to reply to my letters. Common courtesy should have dictated that his recognition of Dr. Hunter's contribution to Canadian agriculture be made at our reunion. His letter dated July 11, 2001, follows:

Mrs. June Hunter

Dear Mrs. Hunter:

I am writing to you at this time regarding the role that your husband, the late Dr. Harold Hunter, played in the 1952 foot-and-mouth (FMD) outbreak in Saskatchewan following his graduation from the Ontario Veterinary College (OVC) in 1951.

Recent outbreaks of FMD in Europe and South America have demonstrated that a disease such as this can enter any country regardless of the preventative measures in place. Today, as in 1952, Canada relies on its veterinary and farming communities, not only to help prevent the entry of exotic diseases, but also to raise awareness of the potential devastation that such a disease outbreak would have for all Canadians. Veterinarians are often the first to report the appearance of disease, thereby enabling emergency measures to be mobilized. They must respond quickly and decisively to limit the spread of disease and the effects that such outbreaks can have on Canada's economy.

We can only speculate on what could have happened to our agricultural industry in 1952 had it not been for the dedicated role played by Dr. Hunter in the detection and subsequent eradication of FMD in Saskatchewan. The fact that Dr. Hunter was able to diagnose FMD, based solely on what he had learned as an OVC student, showed his conviction and personal confidence. His ability to diagnose this exotic disease also underlines the quality of veterinary education in Canada. Today's generation of veterinarians, using the tools of excellence built by their predecessors, can make similar valuable contributions to Canada's continuing prosperity.

As Minister of Agriculture and Agri-Food, and on behalf of all Canadians, please accept my sincere appreciation for the role that your husband played in the 1952 FMD epidemic in Saskatchewan. I am certain that you and your family are very proud of him.

Yours sincerely
Lyle Vanclief

I decided to attempt to obtain suitable recognition by the government of Canada for Dr. Hunter's outstanding contribution. I wrote the following letter to the Minister of Agriculture with the hope that he could facilitate proper recognition. I had hoped that should he answer, his reply could be included in my memoirs. I followed the letter to the Minister with an e-mail telling him that I anticipated that my memoirs would be ready for publication on September 10, 2002. As of that date there had been no answer. His failure to respond convinces me that the federal government is still unwilling to admit their fiasco of fifty years ago. It seems to me that the cost of admitting the mistake and the cost of a suitable posthumous award would be negligible. Such recognition by the government of Canada would have formed excellent public relations for them and would have been appreciated by the veterinary profession, by the producers of livestock, and by the taxpayers of this country. Rather than act on a matter such as this, the Liberal government prefers to advertise by means of very expensive boondoggles such as their sponsorship of hunting and fishing shows in Quebec, currently being investigated by the RCMP.

August 14, 2002

The Honourable Lyle Vanclief
Minister of Agriculture
Ottawa, Ontario
K1A 0C5

Dear Mr. Vanclief

In my last letter to you I asked you to recognize the contribution made by Dr. Harold Hunter with respect to his 1951 diagnosis of foot-and-mouth disease in Saskatchewan. I had hoped that you would make an effort to recognize this contribution at the 50th anniversary of our graduation from the Ontario Veterinary College.

I am completing the final revision of a book entitled The Autobiography Of A Veterinarian. *It is a story of my life and includes a chapter on FMD. Copies of some of my correspondence are included as well as a copy of your letter to Mrs. Hunter dated July 11, 2001, that she kindly provided to me. I had hoped that your letter to her could have arrived in time to be read at our anniversary proceedings. Unfortunately it was too late for presentation at our con-*

cluding meeting. A copy of this letter to you will be included in my memoirs as well as of your reply should such be received prior to publication, which is estimated to be four to six weeks from now. I will be pleased to include you as one to receive a complimentary copy, should you so request.

Recently the Department of Agriculture in Britain acknowledged that the delay in measures to control the recent outbreak of FMD in that country was responsible for substantial excess costs to their economy. The government of Canada with respect to the 1951-1952 outbreaks in this country should admit the same thing. Such an admission could help to alert the public about the economic cost of the disease.

Both the federal government veterinarians and the veterinarians in the employ of the province of Saskatchewan disputed Dr. Hunter's clinical diagnosis. It was not until Dr. Carlson, an employee of the Saskatchewan government, broke the then existing federal rules by submitting samples to the federal government laboratory in Hull that the true nature of the disease was known. When these samples were examined, the clinical diagnosis by Dr. Hunter was confirmed. This confirmation was some three months after the clinical diagnosis.

Your letter to Mrs. Hunter alluded to the eradication of the disease in 1952. No mention was made of the three-month hiatus between the clinical diagnosis and its confirmation. Furthermore, the then Health of Animals Division of the Department of Agriculture by some means lost the paperwork related to Dr. Hunter's contribution. I talked to someone in your department who told me that there was no record of a Dr. Hunter having any part in the outbreak of the disease. I advised him that the newspaper archives of both the Regina Leader Post and the Guelph Mercury contained accounts of Hunter's participation. Suddenly, when their research was done, it was agreed that he was in fact the veterinarian who had stuck by his diagnosis, which in my opinion is the most important diagnosis ever made by a Canadian veterinarian.

I believe that the government of Canada should recognize his contribution to the livestock industry and to the economy of the country. The following suggestions are submitted for your consideration.

1. A posthumous award such as the Order of Canada could be made for his contribution to the country. Canada has made many such awards to a variety of people who were much less deserving of recognition.

2. The government of Canada has made historical awards for unique accomplishments. Canada made this award to the descendants of Igor Gouzenko for his contribution during the cold war.

Recently an old diary written by Dr. Hunter during the foot-and-mouth outbreak has been discovered. While I have not read his accounts of the problem, I have been told that it contains a day-to-day recital of some of his experiences. The suggestion has been made to Mrs. Hunter that she should donate this unique volume to the National Archives in Ottawa and reproductions of it be made for the veterinary colleges in Canada. I have advised Mrs. Hunter that this would be a wonderful contribution to Canada. It is my hope that the government of Canada will contribute by making a suitable award to accompany this volume in its place in Canada's history.

Yours truly

J.E.B. Graham DVM

Copies to:
Mrs. June Hunter
Dr. Alan Meek, Dean, Ontario Veterinary College

As of March, 2004, there has been no reply to this letter.

Chapter Forty-Three

The Need for Vigilance

Agroterrorism is a new word, not yet included in the dictionaries or word processors of the English language. Nor, thankfully, has it yet become a fact. But any discussion of a pandemic livestock or crop disease opens this frightening topic.

In the late 1950s a budding author named Arthur Hailey was our neighbour. His first novel, *Flight into Danger,* had become a best-seller. Arthur and his wife Sheila were clients of mine and attended various local functions as we did. He and I often discussed a variety of topics. One day we got on the subject of foot-and-mouth disease, in which he exhibited a good deal of interest. He thought that this topic could be the basis of a novel based on a bad guy acquiring the virus with the intent of spreading it across North America. This act of sabotage would decimate the livestock industry and result in economic chaos. I agreed that his novel would be fascinating to read but would have the potential of moving some demented person to actually execute the idea set out in his book. He was dissuaded from writing this novel.

295

Today we face another era where terrorism seems to be rampant. It is likely that dissemination of this disease would be a consideration for terrorist activity. I have made several attempts to have one of the Canadian newspapers write a factual and complete series of articles on FMD to educate readers on the inherent economic danger it poses. So far there has been little interest in publishing such a series.

On January 28, 2002, the *National Post* newspaper ran an article by Margaret Munro suggesting that North America is not ready for agroterrorism. While the plot is fictional, the article demonstrates how rapidly the disease could be spread, either intentionally or by accident. She quotes several respected authorities. One of these, Dr. Corrie Brown, a veterinary pathologist at the University of Georgia who has spent plenty of time contemplating such horrors, estimates that an outbreak of the disease could cost the United States $27 billion US. At a conference in Toronto she stated, "It is about economic destruction." As well as foot-and-mouth disease, she listed other animal diseases, such as hog cholera and avian influenza, that could have the potential for economic disaster. She is not worried about giving ideas to the terrorists. She states that they already know their stuff.

Canadian veterinarians agree with the threat and the need to prepare. Dr. Lorne Babiuk, specialist in animal vaccines at the University of Saskatchewan, said that if you get a hit of foot-and-mouth disease or avian influenza, the impact could bring a country to its knees economically.

Munro also states (and this statement is widely known) that Agriculture Canada does not consider animal disease research to be a priority and spends much more on crops than it does on animals. As of early 2000, all of the four veterinary colleges in Canada are rundown and are in danger of losing their accreditation from the international body that ensures the standards of these colleges. The federal government has been asked for $180 million dollars to upgrade their facilities. Some funds were provided after 2001, but more funding is still necessary.

Chapter Forty-Four

A Most Unusual
Veterinarian

When one becomes a senior citizen, some things increase in importance, one of which is the necessity to see old friends at least one more time. I phoned my former preceptor Dr. Bill Steinmetz to find out if a visit would be convenient. I was pleased when he replied that I would be made welcome. My flight from Toronto to Sacramento, California, was booked for November 7, 2003, and the visit was to last until November 11, when I would return to Tampa, Florida, near our winter residence.

Both Bill and his wife Janis are eighty-eight years old and have been married for thirty-eight years. Each has a family from previous marriages; Bill with a son and daughter, and Janis with a son and daughter as well. She had two daughters; the younger died three years ago following a heart transplant. This tragedy severely affected her, and there was a strong probability that she would not recover. Bill took over the duties of nurse, cook, housecleaner, grocery shopper, chauffeur, etc., and with his help she has gradually recovered.

I had not seen Bill for more than ten years and looked forward to our visit. He had been mentioned in the first edition of my autobiography, and I wanted to upgrade the data for the revision currently in progress. Bill is reluctant to give information about his accomplishments. He will never sprain his elbow by patting himself on the back.

We sat for two evenings in the office of his home to discuss some of his accomplishments. Gradually I got him to divulge a lot of information, most of which was new to me, even though I have known him since 1949. Because of this new information about him, I would like to share with those who read my revised book some details about a remarkable person.

I knew from my earlier association with him that his clients considered him to have exceptional diagnostic and surgical skills. During this time together, we visited several veterinary practices. A client was leaving one of them as we entered, and she recognized Bill who was her veterinarian some sixteen years earlier before he retired from active practice. She, like so many others in previous years, was eloquent with her praise.

The city of Sacramento formed the first zoological society in the latter mid '50s. The purpose of this society was to support the zoo and assist in all its activities. That would include the obtaining of new animals, when available, and providing adequate quarters, pens, or other enclosures for the display to the public. Efforts were to be made to provide an environment that would be as similar as possible to their natural surroundings.

At that time, Bill was the attending veterinarian of the zoo and Hank Spencer was the curator. Both men served on that first board. Bill, through the local veterinary association, involved several of his colleagues to participate by meeting with a number of young people who, through their fondness of animals, were interested in a career in veterinary medicine as well as other careers. That necessitated monthly meetings with these young people, not only to expose them to veterinarians of various careers, but also to visit the zoo in the company of a veterinarian. One final activity was that of Little League baseball for young boys aged eight through twelve. Bill worked for ten years with those boys. During that time not all talk was of baseball in itself. Winning and losing were mentioned, and the boys were told to be good winners and good losers, to play the game honestly and the best they could, to have fun and make friends, just as they would throughout life.

In an earlier chapter of these memoirs, I referred to Bill's offer of a loan when the costs of our new veterinary hospital exceeded the estimates. Until this meeting I was unaware that he had given financial help to at least six young veterinarians in the Sacramento area. He stressed that all had repaid their loans with interest. During our visit he took me around the city to see these clinics and to introduce me to these young veterinarians. I sensed that all of them had a high regard for their benefactor. One of these young veterinarians, at my request, offered to tutor Bill on how to use a computer. These lessons were started after my visit. Perhaps you can teach an old dog new tricks!

During our evenings together, Bill discussed his work with the California Veterinary Association (CVMA). Until then I was unaware of the work that he had done for this association, and since I believe that my readers will be impressed with his activities, I will review this aspect of his life.

In 1965, he was elected president of the CVMA, an unpaid position. Since he had a lot of ideas to improve the organization, he took six months' leave of absence from his practice and personally paid for professional help to fill in for him. During this period he visited a majority of the veterinary associations in the state (approximately thirty). One of his ideas stressed the importance of continuing education so that members could keep up with advances in professional knowledge. In addition to his travels around the state, he took three courses, Physiology, Radiology, and Small Animal Practice, at the veterinary college in Davis, California, to upgrade his own knowledge.

Because of his active involvement as president, he received the Veterinarian of the Year award from the state of California. This award is given only occasionally, rather than annually, to the outgoing president. The plaque is inscribed:

VETERINARIAN OF THE YEAR AWARD FOR OUTSTANDING SERVICE TO THE VETERINARY PROFESSION

In 1972, Bill was instrumental in setting up a two-year training course for animal health technicians and taught the course for its first year. In 1976, the board of examiners for the state of California (the licensing body for the profession) presented him with an award for the outstanding dedication of his leadership as president and for his efforts in setting up the technician's course in California.

In 1967, he received an award from his home association, the Sacramento Valley Veterinary Medical Association. It is gratifying to be honoured by local colleagues.

In 1982, he received a special award from the CVMA that was called **"The Distinguished Lifetime Membership Award."**

During the latter 1990s, Bill, with several other senior veterinarians, was instrumental in establishing the new CVMA headquarters located at 1400 River Park Drive, Sacramento. This attractive and functional new building features a series of offices for the staff, meeting rooms, boardrooms, computer rooms, kitchen, and a museum displaying old artifacts related to the profession. In addition, these same senior veterinarians began to write a book on the history of the CVMA. The time required for planning and constructing the new offices and for the preparation of a book on the history of the profession in the region was approximately five years, and both were done at the same time. Bill was involved as well with this planning and actively worked on these projects. In 2001, he received another award from the CVMA for this work.

In July 2000, he received the most prestigious award of the CVMA—the Lifetime Achievement Award—inscribed as follows:

THE CALIFORNIA VETERINARY MEDICAL ASSOCIATION BESTOWS ITS HIGHEST HONOR UPON

WILLIAM E. STEINMETZ DVM

IN RECOGNITION OF HIS OUTSTANDING LEADERSHIP, DIRECTION AND EXTRAORDINARY CONTRIBUTION TO THE ADVANCEMENT OF VETERINARY MEDICINE AS WELL AS ORGANIZED VETERINARY MEDICINE

In the more than one hundred years of its existence, this was only the third time that the CVMA had extended this recognition.

I am sure that readers will agree that Bill Steinmetz is a worthwhile model for young veterinarians to emulate. His model of professionalism could be applied to any field of endeavor:

1. One should be a good family man, and this is most important during the illness of a loved one.

2. Be good enough in your profession to earn the respect of your clients and colleagues.

3. Work with the children of the community, and guide them to achieve excellence in their chosen field.

4. Assist young members of your profession. Consider them as colleagues rather than as competitors.

5. Work actively with your local association. The quality of all professional associations depends on the input of the members.

Our health permitting, Bill has agreed to visit me in Ontario during the summer of 2004.

Epilogue

Give it Back Rather Than Take it Away

In his inaugural speech as incoming president of the United States, John Fitzgerald Kennedy said to his audience: "Ask not what your country can do for you; ask what you can do for your country." His words were wise. It is unfortunate that many citizens of his country as well as many citizens of Canada have not followed his advice but rather have done precisely the opposite.

I wrote this story of my life primarily for my granddaughter Caroline. I want to include Joan's grandchildren in these memoirs. In order of birth they are: David Grainger, Charlie and Marie's son. David graduated as an engineer in 2003 and is an outstanding junior bridge player. Nancy and Jim Wilson have three beautiful daughters, Maxine, Adrienne, and Carolyn. Last but not least is Liam, John and Shirley Grainger's son, now six years old. Liam is one of the most intelligent six-year-old children that I have known. Each of these grandchildren has the ability to do well in his or her chosen field. I hope that all of these young people will attain their potential.

Children are the contribution that their parents make to the future and which they in turn must make for mankind. They should be told that everyone makes mistakes and that the important thing to learn from a mistake is that it should not be repeated. They should be nourished on the principle that part of their success in life should be returned in some form to benefit those who may be less fortunate.

During the latter years of my life, I have reflected on what contribution I have made to humanity and what more I could do. As one of the children of a poor farming family, I learned from my parents the meaning and importance of integrity and the necessity to be fair in dealing with friends and associates. This lesson has been an important part of my life and has, in most cases, led to my success in dealing with people.

During my years as a practising veterinarian, my policy was to provide quality veterinary medicine at a fair fee. Most clients were pleased with my management of the many different problems related to the health of their pets.

I felt that I owed a lot to my profession and wanted to do something to repay my debt. I wrote professional papers on a variety of subjects and prepared a series of lectures devoted to numerous aspects of the profession. These papers and lectures were presented in several countries. It would be fair to say that the time and money expended in the preparation of this material substantially exceeded my remuneration.

Subsequent to my years in practice, I entered a new field as real estate consultant and business advisor to the veterinary profession. Since I was the first veterinarian in Canada to enter this business, the new endeavour was needed and appreciated by my colleagues.

As a memorial to my wife of more than forty years, I provided the seed money to start a breast cancer research study. It was entitled the Barbara Graham Breast Cancer Research Project. The funds were equally divided between McMaster University and the University of Guelph. This was the first time that two teaching hospitals, one in human medicine and the other in veterinary medicine, worked together to develop what has turned out to be a wide-ranging cancer research project. While the study shows little application in animal breast cancer, it shows a lot of promise in the treatment of human breast cancer. Other types of cancer, such as malignant melanoma as well as some forms of leukemia, in both humans and animals, have also shown response to the treatment developed at the two universities.

Barbara's and my only child Janet was encouraged to have a career in medicine. She first obtained a Bachelor of Science in Nursing and later a degree in Medicine. She and her husband Michael have a thirteen-year-old daughter Caroline, who is an excellent student. While Caroline has not as yet chosen a career, she has shown advanced mental ability and, provided that her scholastic interests continue, she should be outstanding in whatever field she chooses.

It should be remembered that the primary function of humans, as well as all other animals, is the perpetuation of the species. Thanks to Janet's success in medicine and to Carolyn's potential, it seems that the gift of life given by Barbara and me will be our most important gift to humanity.